Royal Liverpool University Hospital – Staff Library

Please return or renew, on or before the last date below. Items can be renewed twice, <u>if not reserved for another user</u>. Renewals may be made by telephone: 0151 706 2248 or email: <u>library.service@rlbuht.nhs.uk</u>.
There is a charge of 10p per day for late items.

2 5 SEP 2012

2 2 JUN 2009

0 9 OCT 2009

1 6 MAY 2014

1 4 DEC 2009

2 0 JUL 2010

0 1 MAR 2012

MAKING SENSE OF CLINICAL EXAMINATION OF THE ADULT PATIENT

MAKING SENSE OF CLINICAL EXAMINATION OF THE ADULT PATIENT

A HANDS-ON GUIDE

Douglas Model
MBBS BSc (Physiology) FRCP
American University of the Caribbean,
St Maarten, West Indies
Formerly Consultant Physician,
Eastbourne District General Hospital,
Eastbourne, UK

Hodder Arnold

A MEMBER OF THE HODDER HEADLINE GROUP

First published in Great Britain in 2006 by
Hodder Arnold, an imprint of Hodder Education and a member of the
Hodder Headline Group, 338 Euston Road, London NW1 3BH

http://www.hoddereducation.com

Distributed in the United States of America by
Oxford University Press Inc.,
198 Madison Avenue, New York, NY 10016
Oxford is a registered trademark of Oxford University Press

British Library Cataloguing in Publication Data
A catalogue record for this book is available from the British Library

Library of Congress Cataloging-in-Publication Data
A catalog record for this book is available from the Library of Congress

ISBN-10 [normal]: 0 340 928 247
ISBN-13 [normal]: 978 0 340 928 240
ISBN-10 [ISE]: 0 340 928 425
ISBN-13 [ISE]: 978 0 340 928 424
(International Students' Edition, restricted territorial availability)

1 2 3 4 5 6 7 8 9 10

Commissioning Editor: Joanna Koster
Project Editor: Jane Tod
Production Controller: Lindsay Smith
Cover Design: Nichola Smith
Indexer: Shirley May, Indexing specialists (UK) Ltd
Artist: Kate Nardoni
Cover artwork: Barking Dog Art

Typeset in 10½ on 13 pt Rotis Serif by Phoenix Photosetting, Chatham, Kent
Printed and bound in Italy

What do you think about this book? Or any other Hodder Arnold title?
Please visit our website: www.hoddereducation.com

To my wife, Jillie, and to the students who inspired this book. Teaching the students has been both a privilege and a joy.

The more knowledge and the more facts and concepts you have at your immediate disposal, the more use you will be to your patients.

Douglas Model

CONTENTS

PREFACE

This book is intended for students at any stage of their training and for doctors who wish to revise. In writing it, I have had two main aims. The first is to explain in a clear, step-by-step manner how to take a history and examine an adult patient. The second is to explain the principles underlying the various parts of the history and as many aspects of clinical signs as possible, as learning is much easier if one understands underlying principles rather than resorting to rote learning – both, however, are necessary to an extent, as medicine is so complex and full of facts as well as ideas and concepts. Examples of the underlying principles that are explained are the physiology of the radial pulse on pages 60–68, cardiac signs on pages 93–111 and respiratory signs on pages 128–39.

Each chapter covers the examination of a complete body system, for example the cardiovascular system or the musculoskeletal system. To make the text clear and enable the book to be used when actually examining a patient or practicing examination techniques, as well as for private study, most chapters are presented in two parts. First is a clearly labelled *Examination* section consisting of short bulleted paragraphs containing step-by-step details of examination techniques. Following this are *Background* sections consisting of conventional paragraphs containing details of the principles underlying the various signs.

In the hope that students will find them helpful, I have also included clinical vignettes and text boxes containing symptoms and signs and the clinical features of many common conditions such as myocardial infarction and rheumatoid arthritis.

To avoid repeating the terms 'he or she' and 'his or her' many times on the same page, the patient is referred to throughout as if he or she is male, although with the exception of the chapters on the examination of the breasts and genitalia, the text applies equally to patients of both sexes.

Finally, I welcome suggestions for improving this book.

Douglas Model
2006

ACKNOWLEDGEMENTS

I am grateful for the help of many people in the preparation of this book, in particular Dr John Mikuta for advice and correcting the text, Dr Charles Perakis for extending my knowledge of teaching techniques, Dr Ronald Gagne for discussions about making a diagnosis, and Dr Gordon Caldwell for making suggestions about improving the text.

I am also grateful to the following at Hodder Arnold: Clare Weber for supporting me throughout, Dr Carrie Walker for being so patient and allowing me to move large tracts of text from one part of the book to another at the last moment, Liz Weaver for sorting out the mess I made of the proofs, Jane Tod for encouraging and helping me latterly, Kate Nardoni for turning the crude drawings I supplied into such clear fine diagrams, and last but not least, the typesetters Phoenix Photosetting for producing such a splendid tome.

Douglas Model
2006

LIST OF
ABBREVIATIONS

2LICS	second left intercostal space
2RICS	second right intercostal space
BMI	body mass index
COPD	chronic obstructive pulmonary disease
LMN	lower motor neurone
MMSE	Mini Mental Status Examination
JVP	jugular venous pulse
UMN	upper motor neurone
VSD	ventricular septal defect

PRACTICAL CONSIDERATIONS

DRESS

Dress should meet the patient's expectations of you as a doctor. In some hospitals and family practices, it is customary for male doctors to wear a tie; in others, an open neck shirt or other neat attire is the norm. If you wear a tie, make sure it is secure and does not dangle and act as a source of cross-infection between patients. White coats should be worn where that is the custom. All doctors and students should use a deodorant. Fingernails should be short, so as not to hurt the patient when you are examining him. Hair should be trimmed or, if it is long, should be controlled, so as to avoid getting in the way or tickling the patient when you are bending over him.

BEDSIDE PRACTICALITIES

When examining a female patient, a male examiner should be chaperoned by a woman. Female examiners may also wish to be chaperoned by a woman when examining a male.

Wash or disinfect your hands before and after examining each patient. Failure to do so is an important cause of cross-infection.

When examining a patient, always stand on his *right* side (or occasionally in front). Almost never stand on the left side. This is because it is easier for right-handed people to reach across the patient and use their right hand.

Be gentle; avoid causing discomfort during the examination. Should discomfort occur, apologize to the patient and try to identify its cause.

Never embarrass the patient by exposing him unnecessarily. Remember that exposing one's body to a stranger is both threatening and unnatural, with the added implication that, in the medical situation, something serious and life-threatening may be found. Keep the parts of the body that are not being examined covered by a sheet or examination robe.

Don't take the patient by surprise. Ask his permission before touching him or doing anything to him.

When palpating, use your hands as if they are an extension of your brain and 'think' with the pads of your fingers. When using a stethoscope, use your ears as if they are an extension of your brain and 'think' with your ears.

Be aware that, as ordinary men and women, at times all doctors have sexual thoughts about some of their patients. The wise doctor knows this and addresses it in such a manner that propriety is always maintained and the patient can place his complete trust in the doctor.

THE SUBJECTIVE NATURE OF CLINICAL MEDICINE

Most of the signs described in this book are dependent upon subjective impression rather than objective measurement. It is important to recognize this, as well as the fact that it is the exercise of the judgement and skill this requires that renders medicine an art as well as a science, and ensures that it is a never-ending source of interest and fascination.

2

CLINICAL THINKING AND THE DIAGNOSTIC PROCESS

INTRODUCTION

An accurate diagnosis is essential for the prescription of appropriate treatment. The diagnostic process consists of collecting and synthesizing information about the patient and using it to form hypotheses about the cause of the patient's complaint and how it might be dealt with. As more and more information is collected, the number of hypotheses or possible diagnoses usually becomes less until hopefully only one remains: the definitive diagnosis on which appropriate treatment may be based.

The hypotheses that the doctor accepts or rejects are influenced by many factors such as the patient's age, sex, race, past medical history, family history and psychosocial history, the duration of the complaint and the physical examination. For instance, a simple symptom like a cough will have different connotations in different situations. In a 4-year-old boy whose sister has bronchial asthma, a new cough that has been present for 3 months may arouse suspicion of bronchial asthma, whereas in a in a 64-year-old male heavy smoker, the same type of cough may well arouse suspicion of carcinoma of the bronchus.

The duration or natural history of the complaint is also very important. A patient who develops a hemiplegia over a few minutes or up to an hour or so is likely to be suffering from a stroke, whereas a similar hemiplegia developing over a period of several weeks suggests a slowly developing lesion, such as a brain tumour, or less commonly a subdural haematoma or some other upper motor neurone lesion.

In many ways, being a clinician is like being a detective looking for clues that may be used to deduce the villain. To help him or her, the doctor needs a vast array of concepts and facts upon which to draw. He also needs a good sense of judgement if he or she is to pick out the clues that will lead to the villain. This means developing the ability to carefully weigh up and place a value on the various points of the history and physical examination. Apart from having a vast knowledge, nothing is more important to the clinician than a good sense of judgement. In addition, some clinicians are gifted by a sense of intuition, meaning that they can quite often select the correct diagnosis in one inspired step rather than proceeding in the normal deductive step-by-step manner.

Whether a hypothesis is accepted or rejected is helped by *pattern recognition*, that is recognizing patterns of symptoms and signs. Thus, a middle-aged man with a 2 hour history of severe tight substernal pain radiating to the left arm, accompanied by sweating, a low blood pressure and a fourth heart sound, has a *pattern* of symptoms and signs suggestive of myocardial infarction. Similarly, a 70-year-old man who has suffered a right hemiplegia of sudden onset, accompanied by difficulty in speaking, has a *pattern* suggestive of a stroke or cerebral vascular accident.

From this, it follows that, as long as you are flexible and able to take account of unusual presentations, the more patterns you have stored in your mind, the more likely you will be able to make the correct diagnosis. It also follows that the more you have seen, heard and learned, the better a diagnostician you are likely to be. Although it is sometimes difficult to appreciate the relevance of the finer points of biochemistry or remember the more esoteric pathways connected with the metabolism of cells, as the following case history illustrates, everything you learn in medical school and thereafter may come in useful at a later date.

Shortly after being appointed as a new consultant, a physician was asked to see a 24-year-old woman who had experienced a grand mal seizure a few hours after surgery for suspected acute appendicitis. At operation, her appendix had been found to be normal. The patient denied any past history of seizures, and the consultant surgeon in charge of her case and the anaesthetist who had anaesthetized her were unable to explain the seizure, as general anaesthesia sedates the nervous system and is a recognized treatment for intractable epilepsy.

Fortunately, the physician who had been called to see the patient remembered a case he had heard about when he was a medical student. Trawling through his memory, he recalled a 40-year-old woman who had had a seizure following surgery in exactly the same circumstances as the patient he was about to see. None of the senior doctors in the university hospital where he had been studying as a student, including the professor of medicine, had been able to account for the seizure. Only a registrar was able to do so, as he had heard of a similar case a year or so before. His diagnosis, which proved to be correct, was the rare condition of acute intermittent porphyria.

The new consultant remembered this as he examined the 24-year-old patient, and he remembered learning the biochemistry of the condition and the metabolic pathways leading to the formation of δ-aminolaevulinic acid and porphrobilinogen. And because of what he had learned as a student, he was able to say without hesitation that the 24-year-old woman he had been asked to see was suffering from acute intermittent porphyria.

Urine and blood tests confirmed the diagnosis. Subsequently, when he was asked by the surgeon how he had made the diagnosis so quickly, the physician smiled and replied by telling the story he had heard so long before.

UNCERTAINTY IN THE DIAGNOSTIC PROCESS

In most cases, making a diagnosis and deciding upon the appropriate treatment is straightforward. However, in a significant minority, the process is difficult and beset by uncertainty. In part, this is because many patients do not give a textbook description of their disease. Some diseases present in myriad ways, many of which are atypical, even suggesting a different diagnosis from the correct one.

Another reason for the uncertainty associated with some cases is that medicine involves enquiring into an incredibly complex organism in which hundreds of thousands of biological processes are occurring. As a result, it is sometimes impossible for even a skilled clinician to assemble all the information required to make a diagnosis with certainty, or know with certainty what treatment to offer the patient. Experienced clinicians become used to this, and even enjoy it, as it provides a challenge and is one of things that make the practice of medicine so interesting and an art.

Another difficulty that may confound the diagnostic process is the way we organize and classify information in our minds. As a result, we tend to think of diseases as if they are discrete entities or neat packages of symptoms and signs to which diagnostic labels can be attached, whereas in reality they are much more complex and variable in the ways they present and sometimes overlap.

The autoimmune diseases are an example of the way in which diseases may overlap. Polymyalgia rheumatica can develop into classical temporal arteritis, and rheumatoid arthritis can overlap with systemic lupus erythematosus. Indeed, it has been suggested that polymyalgia rheumatica is not a discrete entity but is instead merely part of the spectrum of temporal arteritis. Because of this uncertainty, it is important to be flexible and keep an open mind and to be ready to change one's thoughts if necessary.

The importance of being flexible and not being rigid is amply demonstrated by the following case history.

> *A 22-year-old woman with a 3-day history of jaundice and a 3-week history of pains in the fingers and other joints was admitted from Accident and Emergency by the duty medical registrar, who was part of a gastroenterological team. On examination, the woman was anaemic. A blood count revealed a normocytic normochromic anaemia, a raised reticulocyte count, a low neutrophil count and a low platelet count. The registrar made a provisional diagnosis of arthritis, haemolytic anaemia, leucopenia and thrombocytopenia due to systemic lupus erythematosus, and asked for the appropriate investigations.*
>
> *The following morning, his chief took him to task. Because he was a gastroenterologist with a special interest in liver disease and was a man of rigid preconceived ideas, the consultant thought of jaundice as having only one cause – liver disease. Subsequently, however, the patient developed a butterfly rash over the bridge of her nose, and all the investigations were compatible with systemic lupus erythematosus.*

MAKING A DIAGNOSIS IN EVERYDAY PRACTICE

The diagnostic process is usually divided into three parts: the history, the physical examination, and the laboratory tests and other investigations. The history is the most important of these, as it alone can lead to the diagnosis in up to 80 per cent of general medical outpatients. In addition, it usually yields information that is helpful with the physical examination and the choice of investigations.

Diagrammatically, the diagnostic process may be summarised as shown in Fig. 2.1.

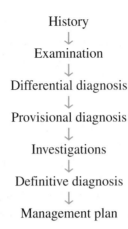

History
↓
Examination
↓
Differential diagnosis
↓
Provisional diagnosis
↓
Investigations
↓
Definitive diagnosis
↓
Management plan

Fig 2.1 The diagnostic process

ORGANIZING YOUR THOUGHTS

In some cases, the pattern of symptoms and signs with which a patient presents is pathognomonic of a single disease, and the diagnosis is easy. In other cases, several alternative hypotheses or diagnoses seem possible. A list of these alternatives is known as the *differential diagnosis.* Up to half a dozen or so of these alternatives should be listed in descending order of likelihood at the end of the history and examination. A list of more than about six or eight suggests that the doctor is uncertain and should think again.

Because it is so common, the symptoms and differential diagnosis of chest pain are listed in Box 2.2 at the end of this chapter.

TIPS ABOUT MAKING THE DIFFERENTIAL DIAGNOSIS

Two important factors to bear in mind when accepting or rejecting hypotheses about possible diagnoses are:

1. Common things happen commonly.
2. Consider the pathology that might account for the patient's history and physical findings.

Common things happen commonly

Common sense dictates that it is sensible to put the most likely diagnoses or hypotheses at the top of the differential list and the rarer ones at the bottom.

Importance of knowing the likely pathology

Making a diagnosis is much easier if you have a good knowledge of the range of pathological changes that occur in a particular tissue, hence the importance to the clinician of having a broad readily available knowledge of physiology, biochemistry, histopathology and microbiology. Doctors who have this and are able to *picture* the histology they are thinking of, or are able to think in terms of the physiology of the system they are dealing with, are much more likely to make a correct diagnosis than those who do not think this way.

As an example, the range of pathological changes that occur in the heart is illustrated in Box 2.1.

Box 2.1: Examples of pathology in the heart

- **Genetic**, e.g. hypertrophic cardiomyopathy (often familial)
- **Congenital**, e.g. atrial or ventricular septal defect
- **Degenerative**, e.g. atherosclerosis of the coronary arteries
- **Neoplastic**, e.g. atrial myxoma
- **Traumatic**, e.g. a knife wound to the pericardium and/or cardiac muscle
- **Endocrine**, e.g. hyperthyroidism causing heart failure
- **Metabolic**, e.g. hypokalaemia or hyperkalaemia causing cardiac arrhythmias
- **Inflammatory/immunological**, e.g. rheumatic fever, Dressler's syndrome
- **Infective**, e.g. viral myocarditis, infective endocarditis
- **Deficiency**, e.g. beriberi due to deficiency of vitamin B_1 (thiamine) causing heart failure
- **Environmental factors**, e.g. smoking causing accelerated atherosclerosis, drugs such as pro-arrhythmic drugs causing cardiac arrhythmias, beta-blocking drugs occasionally causing or worsening heart failure

With an awareness of the different types of pathology that may affect a tissue and an emphasis on the concept that common things happen commonly, you will be in a position to make the next step of the diagnostic process, which is to select the most likely hypothesis or *provisional diagnosis* from the list of the differential diagnoses. After that, the next step is to use the provisional diagnosis to order any investigations that may be appropriate, although in many cases none is needed. As soon as the results of any necessary investigations are available, the final step in the diagnostic process is to amend the provisional diagnosis (if necessary) to arrive at the *definitive (or final) diagnosis.*

PROBLEM-BASED MEDICINE

Apart from making a definitive diagnosis, at this point it is a good idea to list all the other health problems that have come to light during the history, examination and investigation of the patient. This approach is known as *problem-based medicine.* With this list, you will then be able to address both the definitive diagnosis and all the patient's other health problems, and so practise holistic medicine.

For example, the definitive diagnosis and problems needing attention in a 50-year-old man who has suffered a heart attack might be:

● definitive diagnosis: myocardial infarction

● other problems needing attention:
  ○ urgent investigation of hyperglycaemia
  ○ obesity
  ○ osteoarthritis of the right knee
  ○ smoking
  ○ unhappy marriage and impending divorce.

Having made the definitive diagnosis and drawn up a list of the patient's other health problems, you are now in a position to draw up a management plan consisting of the following:

● **Informing the patient** of the diagnosis and discussing the treatment options and actions he can take to optimise his health and increase his longevity, such as stopping smoking, improving his diet and taking more exercise. He should also be informed of follow-up arrangements.

● **General management**, such as referral to a physiotherapist, occupational therapist, dietitian, social worker, priest, cardiac rehabilitation team, etc.

● **Medical management**, such as surgery and/or drug treatment, remembering that to become familiar with the complexities of prescribing drugs, it is a good idea to *write out* the following details of each drug you would prescribe, even if you are a student and not the prescribing doctor in charge of the patient, namely its *generic name*, *dose* and *frequency* and the *duration of the prescription.*

SYMPTOMS AND DIFFERENTIAL DIAGNOSIS OF CHEST PAIN

Box 2.2: Symptoms and differential diagnosis of chest pain

Tip: Think of all the organs in the chest and one or two outside the chest

● **Heart**
　○ *Myocardial infarction*: tight, heavy or constricting central chest pain at rest or persisting after exertion, often radiating to the arm and/or jaw
　○ *Angina*: similar pain to the pain of myocardial infarction, but occurring with exertion or anxiety and relieved by rest
　○ *Pericarditis*: sharp central chest pain worse with deep breathing and lying flat. Eased by sitting upright and leaning forwards

- **Aorta**
  - *Dissecting aneurysm*: tearing pain of abrupt onset moving up to the neck and then down the front or back of the chest as the dissection enlarges

- **Lungs**
  - *Pleurisy*: sharp unilateral pain, worse with coughing and breathing
  - *Spontaneous pneumothorax*: tearing, unilateral pain of abrupt onset
  - *Pancoast tumour*: unremitting severe pain over the top of the shoulder and down the arm
  - *Tracheobronchitis*: raw central chest pain worse with coughing and breathing

- **Oesophagus**
  - *Oesophagitis*, *hiatus hernia*: tight, indigestion-like pain in the centre of the chest, often worse after food or lying flat
  - *Tertiary contractions*: severe tight central chest pain often precipitated by swallowing
  - *Oesophageal rupture*: deep severe central chest pain, usually after vomiting

- **Musculoskeletal system**
  - *Torn muscle fibres*, *osteoarthritis*, *cracked ribs*, *metastases*, *Bornholm disease*: sharp pain worse with breathing, coughing, movement and local pressure

- **Skin**
  - *Herpes zoster (shingles) and post-herpetic neuralgia*: burning pain localized to a dermatome

- **Abdomen**
  - *Referred pain* from a peptic ulcer, biliary colic or subdiaphragm (all of which may also be referred to the shoulder)

- **Psyche (psychological)**
- *Da Costa's syndrome*: pricking or sharp pain over the left breast, lasting seconds or hours without any obvious physical cause

3

HISTORY-TAKING

INTRODUCTION

In the past, doctors tended to be paternalistic and dispense advice, which patients were more or less expected to follow. Now patients are more educated about medical matters and expect to be informed and involved in decisions about their care. As a result, the relationship between the doctor and the patient has become more patient centred, with each party bringing his or her knowledge and point of view to the relationship. The patient knows what he feels, and seeks help from the doctor; the doctor's role is to interpret those feelings in terms of his or her knowledge and offer the appropriate help, which the patient has the right to decline if he wishes without impairing the relationship. One way of thinking of the doctor–patient relationship is to look upon yourself as the patient's advocate and friend, and to treat the patient as you would like to be treated or as you would like a member of your family to be treated.

Essentially, the history is the story of the patient's present complaint, together with such information as his past health and the health of his family. As this involves parting with a lot of personal information and confidences, it places the doctor in a unique position of trust that he or she must respect.

Taking a medical history is both an art and an act of imagination. A good history-taker will obtain more information from a patient in 5 minutes than a poor historian will obtain in half an hour. Part of the art of taking a good history is to imagine that you are either the patient or in the patient's situation, experiencing all that the patient experienced as his complaint unfolded.

Use language the patient will understand, and keep any explanations simple. If the patient uses medical terms such as 'asthma', 'migraine' or 'angina,' explore precisely what he means, as such terms mean different things to different people. For instance, some people use the word 'migraine' to mean any type of headache, whereas others use the word 'angina' to mean breathlessness or indigestion.

The doctor will usually wish to clarify details of the history by asking questions. Such questions should be *open questions*, meaning that they should be couched in such a way that the patient can say what he means without being constrained by the way in which the question is posed. Thus, if a patient is complaining of chest pain, a doctor should not ask, 'Is it sharp or dull?', as that is a *closed question* that allows the patient only two alternatives. Instead, the question should be posed in terms such as, 'Describe the pain to me' or 'Tell me, what does the pain feel like?', as that allows the patient to say what he feels without being constrained by how the question is posed.

The length and content of the history will depend upon the nature of the patient's complaint and the time available to the doctor. Clearly, a case of myocardial infarction or suspected systemic lupus erythematosus warrants a longer history than a common sore throat.

Experience shows that the best results are obtained by taking a broad view and collecting information about the patient as a whole person and not just as someone with a specific complaint. To facilitate this, the history is divided into the following components:

● present complaint

● history of the present complaint

● past medical history

● family history

● psychosocial history

● review of systems.

RECORDING THE PATIENT'S DETAILS

Clinicians vary in the way they record the history and other details of a patient's case. Some write them out by hand; others enter them into a computer. Most clinicians document the present complaint and the history of the present complaint themselves. However, to save time, before the patient is seen, some doctors ask the patient to fill out a form that asks details of his past medical history, his family history, his psychosocial history and a review of systems. Such forms usually contain lists with boxes or lines on which the patient can place a tick and/or state the year of any event. Other doctors ask a nurse or a clerk to take such details before the patient is seen.

If you are writing on sheets of paper, enter the patient's name and case number on every sheet of paper you write on so that there can be no confusion of one patient with another at a later time.

MAKING A START

Shake hands with the patient and introduce yourself by giving your name and saying that you are a medical student. Sit in such a position that your eyes are at approximately the same level as the patient's eyes, as standing looking down at the patient is intimidating.

Learn to observe and listen carefully. To show that you are paying attention, maintain eye contact throughout the interview, and be respectful and never judgemental. Also be *empathetic*, that is, try to understand the patient's feelings and put yourself in his situation; and be *sympathetic*, that is, by your manner and the things you say, *express* understanding and sympathy for the patient's situation. However, although it is important to be sympathetic and empathetic, it is also important to learn to protect yourself from becoming emotionally drained as a result of too much emotional involvement with your patients.

Do not interrupt unnecessarily when the patient is talking. Research has shown that, on average, doctors interrupt every 20–30 seconds.

Ask the patient his name and age. This helps to establish the patient as an individual. If appropriate, ask the patient how he wishes to be addressed. For children and young people, it may be appropriate to use their first name, but most middle-aged and elderly people prefer to be addressed as 'Mr' or 'Mrs'. Never refer to patients by such familiar and derogatory terms as 'dear' or 'darling', or 'grandma' or 'grandpa'.

Explain to the patient that you are going to take his history, examine him and if necessary order some investigations, and that everything he says is in confidence, although with his consent it may be shared with the medical and nursing team looking after him. Also explain to the patient that he may decline to answer any questions he feels are too personal.

DETAILS OF THE COMPONENT PARTS OF THE HISTORY

Present complaint

Ask the patient why he has come to see you by posing an open question such as, 'Can you tell me what you have come to see me for?' or 'Can you please tell me what you are complaining of?' The way in which such questions are asked is a matter of style that varies from doctor to doctor, and eventually you will develop your own style.

The present complaint is usually a one- or two-line statement, the purpose of which is to introduce and focus the mind on what follows. Typically, the present complaint contains a very short statement of the patient's main problem and its duration, such as 'Chest pain, present 3 hours' or 'Increasing breathlessness, 4 days'.

History of the present complaint

This is usually one or two paragraphs in length and should contain a description of the present complaint, including such information as its location, nature, time of onset, duration, whether it is getting better or worse, what makes it better, what makes it worse, a list of medications, if any, that have been taken for it, and a note of any associated symptoms such as feelings of weakness, sweating or vomiting.

As far as possible, the history of the present complaint should be recorded using the patient's own words, although this need not be verbatim. For instance, the doctor should not alter or interpret the patient's story by recording it in medical terms. If a patient says he has a pain in the centre of his chest on walking, the doctor should not write, 'patient complaining of angina', as to do so might introduce a bias and possibly lead to an incorrect diagnosis.

Encourage the patient if he hesitates or falters by summarising what he has said so far, as it will encourage him by showing that you have been paying attention, and will allow him to gather his thoughts or correct you if necessary.

When the patient has finished giving the history of the present complaint and you have checked what he has said, check that you have all the relevant information by asking a question such as 'Is there anything else you wish to tell me or that I should know?' After that, you may wish to clarify some points by asking a few direct or closed questions. Pain is a good example of the type of problem about which the doctor may wish to ask such questions. The correct diagnosis of the cause of a pain is more likely to be made by asking the questions contained in Box 3.1.

Box 3.1: Questions to ask about a pain

- Where is it? (Location)
- How long has it been present? (Duration)
- What does it feel like? (Character)
- How bad is it? (Severity)*
- How often does it occur? (Frequency)
- How long does it last? (Duration)
- Is it getting better or worse? (Change)
- What makes it better? (Relieving factors)
- What makes it worse? (Aggravating factors)
- Does it move anywhere in your body? (Radiation)
- What were you doing when it first came on? (Initiating factors) – particularly important in pain caused by trauma or the musculoskeletal system

*A subjective impression of the severity of a pain may be obtained by asking the patient how severe the pain is on a scale of 0 to 10, where 0 is no pain and 10 is the severest pain the patient can imagine

---

Knowing which questions to ask is important in the diagnosis of many complaints other than pain. For example, if a patient is complaining of diarrhoea, the doctor will wish to ask some or all of the questions contained in Box 3.2.

Box 3.2: Questions to ask about diarrhoea

- How many times a day is the diarrhoea occurring?
- How long has it been present?
- A description of the stool. What is it like?
- The colour of the stool (an open question)
- Whether there is any blood or slime in the stool (a closed question designed to elicit specific information)
- Whether the stool is ever black (also a closed question designed to find out whether there is blood in the stool, as blood from the upper part of the gastrointestinal tract turns black as it is digested and passes through the bowel)
- Does anyone else you know have diarrhoea? (*Salmonella* infection, for instance, is contagious)
- When did you last travel abroad? (as *Salmonella*, *Escherichia coli*, *Giardia lamblia*, cyclospora and other infections may be acquired abroad)

Enquiring into hidden emotions

Most patients are willing to talk about physical symptoms, such as pain or breathlessness, but find it more difficult to express feelings about emotions, such as anger, fear, jealousy, anxiety, depression or stress that may be contributing to or even causing their physical symptoms. For instance, the patient may not recognize that the headache or the indigestion or breathlessness he is complaining of is a physical manifestation of such an emotion. The importance of hidden emotions is illustrated by the following two case histories.

A 60-year-old woman with a history of occasional migraine experienced a severe exacerbation of her condition associated with such severe headaches each day over a 6-week period that she was eventually referred to a neurologist. Simply talking to the neurologist resolved her symptoms, and in retrospect she reported that she realized the headaches were related to unrecognized stress caused by uprooting her home and moving to a new home in a different part of the country.

A 39-year-old happily married father of three presented with a 2-month history of headaches, pains in the chest, palpitations and feelings that he might die if he continued to jog. The first doctor he saw ordered an electrocardiograph and a computed tomography scan of his head. A second doctor took a more detailed history and uncovered the facts that the patient worked a 60-hour week and was under a lot of stress. Explanation and a slight adjustment of the patient's working week completely resolved his symptoms and enabled him to jog again.

One way of finding out about hidden emotions is to take any opportunity that presents during the course of the history. During the psychosocial history, for instance, when asking about the patient's occupation, it is a good idea to also ask how he feels about it, and if he has a boss and it seems appropriate, how he gets on with him or her. Similarly, if the patient is married and you think it is relevant to the patient's condition and will not cause offence, it may be helpful to ask how he feels about his marriage. You will be surprised by some of the answers you get! Similarly, if the patient has children, and you think it is appropriate, it may be helpful to ask how he gets on with them. A follow-up question that is worth remembering to ask, as it may yield further information, is 'Tell me more about that'.

Past medical history

The purpose of the past medical history is to document the general health of the patient and to identify any condition or conditions, such as diabetes or hypertension, that may be contributing to the present complaint by way of complications.

Start the past medical history by asking about childhood illnesses, such as measles or mumps, and, in addition, the year in which any serious illness, hospitalization, operation or other significant health event occurred. Alternatively, you can ask the patient's age when each incident happened or, if the condition is still present, how long he has had it.

The past medical history should also include details of immunizations (including tetanus), medications and allergies. Patients should be asked to bring their medications with them, so that a list may be made that includes the name of each drug, its dose, its frequency and how long the patient has been taking it.

For example, the past medical history of a 50-year-old man might be:

● German measles aged 4

● chicken pox aged 8

● appendicectomy aged 17

● gonorrhoea aged 21

● diabetes controlled by diet for 7 years

● hypertension for 5 years

● *immunizations*: all childhood immunizations; tetanus 5 years ago

● *allergies*: nuts and bee-stings

● *medications*:
  ○ atenolol 50 mg daily for 5 years
  ○ hydrochlorothiazide 25 mg daily for 5 years
  ○ syringe of adrenaline in case of bee-sting.

Note the way in which each item above is listed to make reading it easy, rather than writing it in a long continuous paragraph that is difficult to comprehend. Listing items under one another is also the clearest way of recording the family history, the psychosocial history and the review of systems.

An alternative way of obtaining the past medical history is for the doctor to use a checklist of diseases that he or she can either ask themselves, or the patient can fill in before he sees the doctor (see, for example, the following checklist box).

✔ checklist

Please state your age or the year when you had any of the following:

Childhood conditions

Measles	☐	German measles	☐	Mumps	☐	Whooping cough	☐
Chicken pox	☐	Scarlet fever	☐	Asthma	☐	Hay fever	☐
Rheumatic fever	☐	Diphtheria	☐	Accidents	☐	Polio	☐
Allergies (specify)	☐			Broken bones		Immunizations:	☐
						Childhood: Yes/No	
						Last tetanus............	

Adult conditions

High blood pressure	☐	Emphysema	☐	Broken bones	☐	Thyroid disorder	☐
Diabetes	☐	Heart failure	☐	Varicose veins	☐	Hepatitis	☐
High cholesterol	☐	Heart attack	☐	Migraine	☐	Venereal disease	☐
Asthma	☐	Stomach ulcer	☐	Stroke	☐	Prostate problem	☐
Chronic bronchitis	☐	Arthritis	☐	Epilepsy	☐	Cancer	☐
				Nervous/mental problem	☐	Other	☐

Operations

Appendix	☐	Hernia	☐	Caesarean section	☐	Cancer	☐
Tonsils	☐	Haemorrhoids	☐	Prostate	☐	Other	☐
Gallbladder	☐	Breast	☐	Varicose veins	☐		

Family history

The purpose of the family history is to establish whether the patient is suffering from an illness passed from one generation to another, and also to establish the longevity and cause of death of the patient's relatives. To this end, details should be collected of the age, illnesses or cause of death of the patient's parents, siblings and children, and also, if time permits, the grandparents and uncles and aunts. One way of starting the family history is to say something such as 'Now I wish to ask about your family history. Can you please tell me if there are any illnesses passed from one generation to another in your family, such as cancer, high blood pressure or diabetes?'

When you have gathered this information, proceed by asking about the health of individual members of the family by saying something such as 'Can you please tell me about your parents [or grandparents] on your father's side? Are they alive, and if so, how old are they and how is their health?' On hearing of the death of a close relative of the patient, it is good practice and common humanity to make a brief expression of sympathy.

An example of the family history of a 50-year-old man might be:

● details of paternal grandparents unknown

● maternal grandfather died of cancer of the bowel aged 84

● maternal grandmother died of heart failure aged 76

● father died of heart attack aged 71

● mother alive and well aged 78, but has high blood pressure, and diabetes controlled by diet

● two brothers aged 45 and 48 alive and well; another brother died in a road accident aged 24

● one son aged 22 had asthma till aged 14; a daughter aged 24 has eczema.

An alternative way of presenting the family history is to record it in the form of a family tree or pedigree (Fig. 3.1).

Psychosocial history

The purpose of the psychosocial history is to collect information about factors in the patient's environment and lifestyle that might be affecting his health and also to collect information about any social needs or support he may have. To this end, information should be collected about the patient's relationships, occupation, occupational hazards, housing, hobbies, habits such as smoking, alcohol intake and use of recreational drugs and, if appropriate, foreign travel.

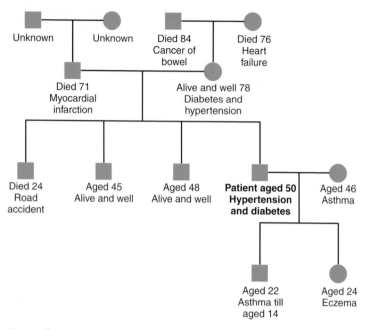

Fig 3.1 Family tree of the 50-year-old man referred to in the text

The importance of asking these questions is amply demonstrated by the following case history.

A 32-year-old woman was referred to the outpatient department with a 3-month history of breathlessness on minor exertion and was seen by a medical registrar who sent her for a chest X-ray, which showed abnormal shadowing at the apices of both lungs. The registrar made a provisional diagnosis of cancer of the lung and referred the patient to a chest physician for bronchoscopy.

Before he bronchoscoped her, the chest physician reviewed the X-rays and decided to ask the patient about her occupation and hobbies. In reply to a question about keeping birds, the patient said, 'No, doctor, I don't keep any birds, but my husband keeps two hundred pigeons at the bottom of the garden.' On hearing this, the chest physician revised the diagnosis to bird fancier's lung and asked for blood to be taken for antibodies against avian proteins (avian precipitins). The result was strongly positive, and as a result the patient was advised that her husband should get rid of the birds. In addition, she was given a short course of oral corticosteroids to which she responded with a complete resolution of her symptoms.

One way of starting the psychosocial history to say something such like 'Now I would like to ask about some background factors in your life. Can you please tell me if you are married, and if not, whether you live with somebody or live on your own?' Depending upon the answer, you may feel it appropriate at this juncture to seek information about hidden emotions in the way described on page 19.

It is important to be able to talk easily to patients about their sex life, particularly if the patient has had a serious illness such as a heart attack, as the patient and/or his partner may be afraid to have intercourse after such a serious event. One way of approaching this is to do so when asking the patient about his relationships. Thus, if the patient is married (or lives with a partner) and the doctor thinks that it is relevant and will not cause offence, it is reasonable to ask a question such as 'Do you and your wife [or partner] make love?' or 'Are you sexually active?' Another less direct way of asking about a patient's sex life is to say something along the lines of 'Are you happy with your sex life?', although this is less likely to yield specific information than a question that asks specifically about it.

In addition, some doctors like to take a spiritual history if they think it might be helpful and relevant. But be careful about this, as the term 'spiritual history' implies something very personal and much more all-embracing than merely asking whether the patient believes in God and follows a religion. In essence, the question involves talking about such all-embracing subjects as one's personal values and the relationship between one's finite mortal self and the infinite immortal scheme around us, and as people do not often talk about such things, the patient may be reluctant to answer. Thus, although knowing the spiritual history may be helpful in some cases, doctors in general are divided about the wisdom of routinely asking about it. However, all agree that a doctor must never use his or her privileged position as a platform from which to impose or seek to impose his or her spiritual views on the patient.

With this reservation in mind, the psychosocial history of a 50-year-old man might be as follows:

- **Relationships:** Happily married for 22 years. Sex life satisfactory. (Or alternatively, if the patient is gay: Gay, in a stable relationship, 10 years.)

- **Occupation:** Lawyer in a group practice.

- **Occupational hazards:** Nil. (*Note:* If appropriate, it is important to ask about exposure to occupational hazards such as asbestos, flour, silage, detergents, etc.)

- **Housing:** Own townhouse with three flights of stairs. (*Note:* Knowing about stairs is important if the patient is suffering from a cardiac or respiratory disease or has a problem with mobility.)

- **Pets:** Keeps a dog and a cat. (*Note:* Knowing about pets is important, as they can be responsible for certain respiratory diseases such as asthma, bird fancier's lung and psittacosis.)

- **Hobbies:** Goes to the theatre and art galleries. Jogs twice a week, cycles to work, hikes at weekends.

- **Smoking:** 10 cigarettes per day for 20 years; stopped 10 years ago. (Note: If the patient is a current smoker, ask about the number of cigarettes smoked per day and the number of years the patient has smoked.)

- **Alcohol:** 3 units per day (where one unit is half a pint of beer, a wine glass of wine or a measure of spirits).

- **Recreational drugs:** Smoked one or two cigarettes of marijuana a month until 10 years ago.

- **Spiritual life:** The patient is a practising Catholic. Says he thinks a lot about the meaning of life and whether there is a life hereafter.

- **Foreign travel:** Holiday in Kenya 3 months ago.

Review of systems

The purpose of the review of systems is to uncover any symptoms that may be contributing to the present complaint and have not been mentioned so far. It is also a means of drawing attention to other conditions that may be important and in need of attention.

Basically, the review of systems involves asking questions about every system of the body. In the box on page 28 is an example of a list of direct questions a patient might be asked. This list is, however, very full, and depending on the doctor's speciality and the pressures of time, the list is in practice often shorter and more focused than the one here. It is suggested that you practise with a list like the one shown here and then formulate a list of your own.

✔ checklist

Please tick or answer as relevant:

General health
Fever ☐
Fatigue ☐
Change of appetite ☐
Weight ☐
  Steady ☐
  Recent gain ☐
  Recent loss ☐

Skin
Rashes ☐
Itching ☐
Suspicious moles ☐
Recent dryness ☐

Ears
Earache ☐
Deafness ☐
Ringing in the ears ☐
Ear discharge ☐
Hearing aid ☐

Mouth and gums
Mouth ulcers ☐
Bleeding gums ☐
Dental problems ☐
Sore throats ☐
Hoarseness ☐

Nose and sinuses
Nose bleeds ☐
Nasal discharge ☐
Nasal obstruction ☐
Sinus pain ☐
Hayfever ☐

Eyes
Long sight ☐
Short sight ☐
Eye pain ☐
Eye discharge ☐
Blurred vision ☐
Double vision ☐
Change of vision ☐

Neck
Stiff neck ☐
Neck pain ☐
Swollen glands ☐
Enlarged thyroid ☐
Lump in the neck ☐

Cardiac
Chest pain ☐
Palpitations ☐
Swelling of ankles ☐
Breathlessness ☐

Respiratory
Cough ☐
Sputum ☐
Breathlessness ☐
Wheeze ☐
Coughing blood ☐

Gastrointestinal
Appetite:
  Good ☐
  Poor recently ☐
    Meat ☐ Fish ☐
    Vegetables ☐ Fruit ☐
Indigestion ☐
Abdominal pain ☐
Difficulty swallowing ☐
Vomiting ☐
Change of bowel habit ☐
Diarrhoea ☐
Constipation ☐
Blood in the stools ☐
Black stools ☐

Urinary

- Pain passing urine ☐
- Frequency: day ☐ night ☐
- Urgency ☐
- Hesitation ☐
- Poor urinary stream ☐
- Past infection ☐
- Blood in urine ☐
- Urinary stones ☐

Genital (male)

- Penile discharge ☐
- Sores on penis ☐
- Testicular pain ☐
- Testicular lump ☐
- Prostate problems ☐
- Sexual dysfunction ☐
- Impotence ☐
- Sexual disease ☐
- Exposure to HIV ☐

Reproductive/genital (female)

- Periods: age of onset
- Regular ☐
- Irregular ☐
- Frequency _____ days
- Duration _____ days
- Light ☐ Moderate ☐ Heavy ☐
- Menopause aged _____ years
- Bleeding since menopause ☐
- Vaginal discharge ☐
- Pain on intercourse ☐
- Birth control? Specify
- Number of children
- Number of miscarriages or abortions
- Exposure to HIV or sexual disease ☐

Endocrine

- Thyroid disorder ☐
- Feeling hot ☐
- Feeling cold ☐
- Excessive sweating ☐
- Hot flushes ☐
- Excessive thirst ☐
- Excessive urination ☐

Nervous system

- Dizziness ☐
- Convulsions ☐
- Muscle weakness ☐
- Pins and needles ☐
- Numbness ☐
- Loss of balance ☐
- Loss of memory ☐
- Headaches ☐

Musculoskeletal

- Muscle or joint pain ☐
- Stiffness ☐
- Muscle weakness ☐
- Limitation of movement ☐
- Arthritis ☐
- Leg cramps ☐

Peripheral vascular

- Varicose veins ☐
- Clots in veins ☐
- Cold hands and feet ☐
- Calf pain on walking ☐

Haematological

- Anaemia ☐
- Easy bruising ☐
- Easy bleeding ☐
- Blood transfusion ☐

Psychological

- Anxiety ☐
- Depression ☐
- Change of mood ☐
- Insomnia ☐
- Abuse:
  - Physical ☐
  - Emotional ☐
  - Sexual ☐

The importance of the review of systems and the part it can play in what is known as problem-based medicine (page 10) is amply demonstrated by the following case history.

A 60-year-old man was seen and thoroughly examined in the outpatient clinic by a consultant neurologist, and was subsequently admitted to hospital for investigation of unexplained neurological symptoms. On the ward, the history and examination were repeated by the house officer.

Although it had nothing directly to do with the patient's neurological condition, during the review of systems, the house officer asked the patient about his bowels and whether he ever passed any blood rectally. The answer was that, over the past 3 months, the patient had occasionally passed a little blood. Rectal examination was normal, but sigmoidoscopy revealed a carcinoma about 12 cm above the anus.

When the consultant was told about the tumour, he wondered momentarily how he had missed it, but then congratulated the house officer on his clinical acumen. Subsequently, the patient was found to be suffering from an unusual form of multiple sclerosis. This bore no relationship to the tumour, which was successfully resected a few days later.

4

GENERAL APPEARANCE OF THE PATIENT

EXAMINATION

- Begin to assess the patient as a whole person from the moment you see him for the first time as he walks in through the door of your office, or from the moment you first see him on a ward or home visit, as the impact he makes and the things you notice about him are likely to be greatest on first acquaintance, before you have become accustomed to him.

- Below is some of the information that may be gleaned from such observations:

- The patient's **manner** and gait, and the way he conducts and holds himself: These parameters provide important clues about both the patient's mental and physical states, and are an important source of information about non-verbal communication. For instance, a patient who holds himself erect and looks happy is probably happy and well (although he may occasionally be harbouring a serious disease), whereas a patient who drags himself in and looks ill is probably physically ill or depressed.

- **Gait**: As he walks, notice the patient's posture and whether he swings his arms. Also note the way he lifts his feet and the way they swing forward and strike the ground. Examples of abnormal gaits are on page 39.

Signs that may be evident on closer inspection

- Is the patient **well** or **ill**?

- Is the patient in **pain** or **breathless**?

- His biological or apparent **age** compared with his calendar or chronological age.

- His state of **nourishment**, and whether it appears to be normal, or whether he is obese or has apparently lost weight.

- His sense of **orientation**, which, if indicated, is easily screened by asking the patient the day of the week and where he is. (The mental status examination for assessing a patient's state of cognition, orientation and memory is on page 156).

- His **mood**, whether for instance he appears to be anxious or depressed, placid or agitated, coherent or confused.

- **Verbal and non-verbal communication**. Clues to this may be obtained by watching the patient's facial expressions and bodily movements, and whether, for instance, he is fidgety or appears to be flushed with anxiety or is depressed.

- **Dress and grooming**. Note whether the patient is neat and tidy, or dishevelled or dirty-looking, and whether he has any tattoos or body piercings or is wearing jewellery.

- **Personal hygiene**. Note any body odours, such as:
  - an unpleasant mouth odour due to poor dentition or chronic sinusitis
  - a smell of alcohol or the stale smell of tobacco
  - the malodour of body odour (BO)
  - a sweet smell of acetone (which may be likened to pear drops), suggesting diabetic ketoacidosis
  - the unpleasant fetid smell of foetor hepaticus, suggesting hepatic failure.

Other signs that may be evident

Cyanosis

- Cyanosis is a blue colouration of the skin and mucus membranes that is assessed by noting the colour of the lips and then asking the patient to show you his tongue and the palmar surfaces of his fingers.

> **Note!**
>
> Background information about cyanosis is on page 40.

Anaemia and jaundice

- While looking at the lips, tongue and hands for cyanosis, also look for paleness resulting from anaemia.

- In addition, look for paleness of the conjunctivae by first explaining to the patient what you are going to do and then gently pulling down both lower eyelids with the tips of your thumbs and inspecting the exposed conjunctivae.

- At the same time as inspecting the conjunctivae, also inspect the sclera for the yellow colour of jaundice, as the sclera are the site at which jaundice usually first becomes visible.

> **Note!**
>
> Background information about anaemia and jaundice is on page 41.

Xanthomata and arcus senilis

While your attention is still on the eye, look for the following:

- **Xanthomata,** which are small yellow deposits of cholesterol 2 or 3 mm in diameter on the skin above and below the nasal side of each eye. Only about 50 per cent are associated with hyperlipidaemia. The other 50 per cent of people with xanthomata on the face have normal serum lipid levels.

- **Arcus senilis,** which is a thin grey ring of lipids deposited in a circle around the periphery of each cornea that looks as if it is around the periphery of the iris. In persons aged less than 60 years, an arcus is a risk factor for atherosclerosis.

Evidence of smoking

- **Smoker's face**: inspect the face for a prematurely worn wrinkled appearance that is a sign of heavy smoking in patients under the age of 70 years. Over the age of 70, the changes are unreliable, as they tend to merge with the changes of old age. About a quarter of heavy smokers have this sign.

- **Nicotine staining**: look for a yellow/brown colour on the index and middle fingers of the hand in which cigarettes are held.

Acromegaly, Cushing's disease or syndrome and adrenal failure

- Inspect the patient for the signs listed in Boxes 4.1–4.3.

Box 4.1: Acromegaly

Due to excess secretion of growth hormone from an acidophilic (eosinophilic) tumour of the anterior pituitary gland

- Hypertrophy of bone and soft tissues causing:
  - ○ Coarse facial features with prominence of the forehead known as *frontal bossing*, enlarged lower jaw known as *prognathism*, a wide long nose, thick lips and a large tongue
  - ○ Large, thick hands and feet
  - ○ Carpal tunnel syndrome
- Excessive sweating and greasy skin
- Bitemporal hemianopia (page 176) due to the tumour pressing on the central nerve fibres of the optic chiasma
- Hypertension
- Impaired glucose tolerance

Box 4.2: Cushing's disease and syndrome

Due to excessive secretion or administration of corticosteroids

- Movement of fat to the centre of the body causing:
  - ○ Round, plethoric moon face
  - ○ Obese trunk and thin legs and arms, i.e. an 'orange on a matchstick appearance'
  - ○ 'Buffalo hump' across the upper back
- Acne and hirsutism due to increased secretion of androgens
- Purple striae on the abdomen due to protein catabolism
- Bruising due to protein catabolism of the vessel walls
- Weakness and muscle wasting due to myopathy (mainly proximal) caused by protein catabolism
- Osteoporosis due to protein catabolism of bone
- Hypertension due to sodium and fluid retention
- Diabetes mellitus
- Confusion and/or psychosis

Note: Simple obesity is differentiated from Cushing's disease or syndrome by the fact that it is associated with obese arms and legs

---

Box 4.3: Adrenal failure (Addison's disease)

Due to failure of secretion of corticosteroids

- Unwellness, malaise, tendency to collapse
- Nausea, vomiting, weakness
- Profound dehydration and electrolyte depletion causing low blood pressure and postural hypotension
- Pigmentation of the buccal mucosa and creases of the hand due to increased secretion of both adrenocorticotrophic hormone and melanocyte-stimulating hormone in patients with primary adrenal failure, but not in cases of primary pituitary failure, in which both are decreased
- Hypoglycaemia
- Typical electrolyte pattern with low serum Na^+ and high serum K^+ due to absence of the sodium-retaining and potassium-losing action of corticosteroids on the distal renal tubule

Hyperthyroidism or hypothyroidism

● Inspect the patient for the signs listed in Boxes 4.4 and 4.5.

> ## Tip
>
> Remember that thyroid hormones control the speed of metabolism and bodily activity.

Box 4.4: Hyperthyroidism

♀:♂::8:1
Goitre in approximately 50 per cent

Fast metabolism and body activity causing:
● Anxiety, irritability
● Fine skin and hair due to catabolism of tissues
● Hot sweaty palms and fine tremor of the hands
● Eye problems in about 50 per cent (ranging from grittiness to exophthalmos)
● Increased appetite
● Weight loss despite increased appetite with or without myopathy (mainly proximal) due to catabolism of proximal muscles
● Sinus tachycardia and bounding pulse
● Fast ankle reflexes
● Atrial fibrillation and/or heart failure in the elderly

Other occasional features
● Lymphocytosis and/or splenomegaly (autoimmune cases)
● Clubbing of the fingers

Box 4.5: Hypothyroidism

♀:♂::8:1
Goitre depending upon cause

Slow metabolism and body activity causing:
- Often no symptoms or signs, *or*:
- Coarse facial features, hoarse voice and carpal tunnel syndrome due to the deposition of myxoedema (mucopolysaccharides) in the face, larynx, tongue and carpal tunnel
- Dry skin, loss of hair and loss of outer eyebrows
- Weight gain
- Mental slowness, depression
- Constipation
- Sinus bradycardia
- Hypercholesterolaemia and angina pectoris in the middle-aged and elderly
- Slow ankle reflexes, particularly the relaxation phase

Other occasional features
- Cerebellar ataxia
- Pleural effusion or ascites

Tremor

Look for one of the three following types of tremor:

- **Resting tremor:** observe the patient as he sits at rest for a continuous rubbing movement between the tips of the thumbs and index fingers that is part of *Parkinson's disease* and is known as a 'pill-rolling' tremor. More exaggerated forms of this type of tremor may involve shaking of the whole hand.

- **Intention tremor:** this is tested for as described on page 204. An intention tremor is present if there is shaking of the fingers and hands on purposeful movements, particularly as the target is approached. An intention tremor is usually an indicator of cerebellar disease (or drunkenness).

- **Fine tremor of the extended hands:** ask the patient to extend the fingers and arms of both upper limbs in a straight line in front of him. A fine tremor may be due to:
  ○ a benign variation of normal – a so-called *essential tremor*
  ○ anxiety
  ○ the after-effect of heavy alcohol intake
  ○ thyrotoxicosis.

- **Liver flap:** ask the patient to hold his fingers and arms straight out in front of him with the hands dorsiflexed. A coarse flap of the extended arms is a sign of liver failure and hepatic encephalopathy.

Dehydration

Inspect the patient for a sunken appearance of the eyes. If the eyes appear to be sunken and you suspect dehydration, look for the following:

- a **sunken appearance of the eyes** and increased space under the eyeballs that is demonstrated by asking the patient's permission and then gently pulling down both his lower eyelids with the tips of your thumbs

- **dryness of the mouth and tongue** demonstrated by asking the patient to open his mouth: a very dry tongue has a dry, leathery appearance

- **abnormal tissue turgor** of the skin at the top of the chest and on the backs of the forearms that is demonstrated by telling the patient what you are about to do, then lifting a fold of skin at the relevant site between your forefinger and thumb, releasing it and observing the time it takes to adopt its normal flat position. This is normally a second or so. With dehydration, it is much longer.

Evidence of hypocalcaemia

Low ionized calcium concentrations increase the excitability of the neuromuscular junction and result in a tendency to involuntary muscle spasms known as **tetany**. If you suspect hypocalcaemia, perform the following tests:

- **Chvostek's sign:** curve the index finger of your dominant hand, and with movements mainly at the wrist, tap the facial nerve (cranial nerve VII) in front of the ear with the tip of the finger. The test is positive if twitching occurs at the corner of the mouth.

- **Trousseau's sign:** place a sphygmomanometer cuff around the patient's upper arm and inflate it to above systolic pressure for 3–4 minutes. The test is positive if spasm of the muscles of the hand occurs with the adoption of a characteristic pose known as *main d'accoucheur*, meaning 'hand of the obstetrician', in which the fingers and thumb are extended and the metacarpal/phalangeal joints are partially flexed.

Background information

Gaits

Normal gait

Normally, the knee flexes, the heel lifts and the arm begins to swing as the patient steps forward. Then, as the step proceeds, the knee straightens, and at the end of the stride, the heel strikes the ground.

Hemiplegic gait

Hemiplegia is paresis of the limbs of one side of the body and is usually due to an upper motor neurone lesion on the opposite side of the brain. Patients with hemiplegia walk with varying degrees of a stiff *flexed arm* and a stiff *extended leg*, which they are obliged to swing out laterally as they walk in order to lift their foot off the ground.

A hemiplegic gait is caused by muscle spasm and the disease process upsetting the balance between the agonist and antagonist muscles. This exposes the fact that, in the arms, the flexor muscles are intrinsically stronger than the extensor muscles, as the main function of our arms is to flex them in order to pull food and other objects towards us, while in the legs the extensor muscles are intrinsically stronger than the flexor muscles, as the main function of our legs is to extend them for standing and walking.

Parkinsonian gait

The three main features of Parkinson's disease are bradykinesia (i.e. slowness and paucity of movements), tremor and rigidity. As a consequence, patients with Parkinson's disease have an expressionless face that lacks movement, and also do not swing their arms. They also often have difficulty with starting to walk, which they do by throwing themselves forward and taking small steps, as if trying to catch up with their centre of gravity in a process known as a *festinant gait.*

Wide-based gait

Patients with incoordination due to cerebellar disease (or drunkenness) usually walk with an unsteady gait and their feet wide apart as they try to steady themselves and prevent themselves from falling.

Stomping neuropathic gait

Patients with severe sensory peripheral neuropathy are sometimes not aware where their feet are and as a consequence lift them high off the ground in what is described as a *stomping gait.*

Foot drop

Patients with dysfunction of the peroneal nerve or the sciatic nerve, which supplies the peroneal nerve, or motor neurone disease may suffer foot drop and drag their foot along the ground as they walk as a result of weakness of the dorsiflexor foot muscles in the anterior compartment of the lower leg that are supplied by the peroneal nerve.

Cyanosis, anaemia and jaundice

Cyanosis occurs when the reduced haemoglobin level in the blood is over 50 g/L, the oxygen saturation of arterial blood is less than 85 per cent or the oxygen tension of the arterial blood is below 10.6 kPa. Two types of cyanosis are recognized: central and peripheral.

Central cyanosis is blueness of the lips and tongue owing to failure of oxygenation of the blood in the lungs as a result of heart disease or lung disease.

Peripheral cyanosis is blueness of the hands and feet, either as part of central cyanosis or as a result of a greater than normal extraction of oxygen from the blood in the periphery due to vasospasm occurring as part of the physiological response to cold. Raynaud's disease and Raynaud's phenomenon are extreme variations of this. Raynaud's disease is a *primary* condition that occurs mainly in otherwise healthy women and is associated with severe vasospasm causing the fingers to turn blue and then white in response to the even modest cold; ulcers or gangrene may occasionally occur. Raynaud's phenomenon is clinically similar but is *secondary* to diseases such as scleroderma and systemic lupus erythematosus.

Anaemia and jaundice

The symptoms of severe anaemia include fatigue, palpitations and breathlessness on exertion, and angina of effort in certain circumstances. Four main types of anaemia are recognized – deficiency, haemolytic, bone marrow failure and chronic illness. Three types of jaundice are recognized – prehepatic (haemolytic), hepatic (hepatocellular) and posthepatic (obstructive).

THE HANDS

Examination

Ask the patient to show you *both* his hands with his wrists and fingers extended, and then use the following checklist to examine both hands from the back and then from the front. Details of the items on the checklist are discussed in the subsequent paragraphs.

✔ checklist for examination of the hand

Back of the hand	Palmar surface of the hand
Occupation	Occupation
Nicotine staining	Anaemia
Arthritis	Cyanosis, Raynaud's disease/ phenomenon
Clubbing of the fingers	Quincke's sign
	Sweaty palms
Nails:	Dupuytren's contracture
Personal care, anaemia, splinter haemorrhages, pitting, white nails, yellow nails, koilonychia	Palmar erythema
	Marfan's syndrome
	Down's syndrome
Neuropathy:	Osler's nodes
Wasting of the interosseus muscles	Neuropathy:
	Wasting of the thenar, hypothenar and interosseus muscles

Background information

Occupation

Rough, worn hands suggest a manual occupation or hobby.

Smoking

Smoking often causes a brown discolouration of the skin, usually on the index and middle fingers of the hand in which cigarettes are held.

Arthritis

Osteoarthritis

Osteoarthritis causes non-symmetrical swelling and deformity of the joints of the knuckles and fingers that is due to the wear and tear associated with age and/or manual occupation. *Heberden's node* is typical of the condition and is an osteophyte (bony outgrowth) on the terminal interphalangeal joint of the index and/or middle fingers of the dominant hand.

Rheumatoid arthritis

In the hands, rheumatoid arthritis causes changes that are typically both *symmetrical* and *bilateral*, and in severe cases results in swelling and subluxation (partial dislocation) of:

- the wrist joints

- the fingers at the metacarpal/phalangeal joints, where there is also usually *ulnar deviation*

- other changes are described in Box 4.6 (page 44), including *spindling* due to swelling of the interphalangeal joints, and *swan-neck deformity*, in which there is hyperextension of the proximal interphalangeal joint and flexion of the distal interphalangeal joint, as demonstrated in Fig. 4.1.

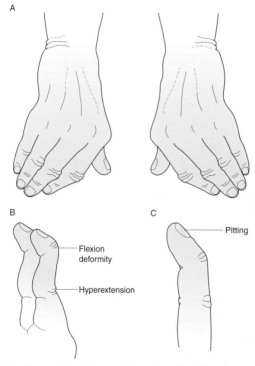

Fig 4.1 (A) Swelling, subluxation and ulnar deviation (B) Swan-neck deformity (C) Psoriatic deformity

The clinical features of rheumatoid arthritis are listed in Box 4.6.

Note!

The subluxation, ulnar deviation and swan-neck deformities described above are the result of the prolonged abnormal pull of muscles and diseased tendons on inflamed joints.

Box 4.6: Clinical features of rheumatoid arthritis

A systemic autoimmune disease of connective tissue mainly affecting serosal surfaces, in particular, the synovial membranes of joints

- Malaise, tiredness, depression and occasionally anorexia, weight loss and pyrexia
- Morning stiffness
- Arthritis
- *Hands*: classically swelling, subluxation and ulnar deviation of the metacarpal/phalangeal joints
- *Swan-neck deformity* of the fingers, i.e. hyperextension of the proximal interphalangeal joints and flexion of the distal interphalangeal joints; *spindling*, i.e. swelling of the proximal interphalangeal joints
- *Feet*: collapse of the foot arch, subluxation of the metatarsal/phalangeal joint and hallus valgus with bunion formation
- *Neck*: atlantoaxial subluxation ± spinal chord compression with numbness and upper motor neurone weakness of the hands and feet
- *Other joints*: arthritis of many other joints, particularly the wrists, knees, ankles and hips
- *Extra-articular manifestations*: rheumatoid nodules on extensor surfaces, episcleritis/scleritis in the eye (red inflammatory lesions on the sclera), anaemia, carpal tunnel syndrome, pleural effusion, interstitial lung disease, dry eyes (keratoconjuctivitis due to Sjögren's syndrome), pericarditis, vasculitis leading to ischaemia and ulcers/gangrene

Systemic lupus erythematosus

This usually results in a non-deforming arthritis, although in some cases it may result in a deforming arthritis similar to rheumatoid arthritis. The clinical features of systemic lupus erythematosus are listed in Box 4.7.

Box 4.7: Clinical features of systemic lupus erythematosus (SLE)

A multi-system autoimmune disease of connective tissue may present with a spectrum of features ranging from an indolent non-specific illness with fatigue to a serious illness with any of the following:

- **Red erythematous malar rash**
- **Red discoid rash**
- **Photosensitivity**

(*Note*: As a result of the above three criteria, the skin is involved in over 75 per cent of cases)

- **Oral ulcers**: usually painless
- **Arthritis**: mainly small joints. Usually non-erosive and non-deforming, but may occasionally resemble rheumatoid arthritis
- **Serositis**: inflammation of the pleura and/or pericardium
- **Renal disease**
  - Proteinuria > 0.5 g/day
  - Glomerulonephritis, ranging from minimal change to crescent forming. Occasionally nephrotic syndrome
- **Neurological**: seizures or psychosis. Also occasionally stroke, cranial nerve palsy or polyneuropathy
- **Haematological**
  - Haemolytic anaemia
  - Neutropenia, lymphopenia or thrombocytopenia
- **Immunological**
  - LE cells, IgG antibodies to double-stranded DNA, or against Ro and La antigens. False-positive syphilis test
- **Anti-nuclear factor antibody** positive in the absence of drugs that can cause positivity, such as hydralazine, methyldopa and isoniazid

Psoriasis

Psoriasis is occasionally associated with a flexion deformity of the *distal* phalangeal joints, as demonstrated in Fig. 4.1.

Clubbing of the fingers (and often the toes)

Mild clubbing is characterized by loss of the normal angle between the proximal part of the nail and the skin overlying the nail bed, as demonstrated in Fig. 4.2. Well-developed clubbing is associated with abnormal expansion of the nail and terminal part of the digit, as demonstrated in Fig. 4.2. Clubbing is associated with the conditions listed in Box 4.8 and, despite what is sometimes said, is of unknown aetiology.

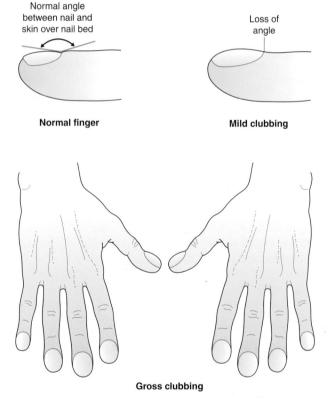

Normal angle between nail and skin over nail bed

Normal finger

Loss of angle

Mild clubbing

Gross clubbing

Fig 4.2 Clubbing of the fingers

> **Box 4.8: Diseases associated with clubbing of the fingers**
>
> - **Chronic pulmonary sepsis**, e.g. tuberculosis, empyema (pus in the pleural cavity), bronchiectasis (localized abnormal dilatations of the bronchi), lung abscess
> - **Carcinoma of the lung** (5 per cent of cases)
> - **Cryptogenic fibrosing alveolitis**, also known as idiopathic pulmonary fibrosis (70 per cent of cases)
> - **Extrinsic alveolitis** due to inhaled organic dusts, e.g. farmer's lung
> - **Inhaled inorganic dust**, e.g. asbestos
> - **Cystic fibrosis**
> - **Cyanotic heart disease**, mainly as a result of right-to-left shunts caused by pulmonary hypertension (Eisenmenger syndrome)
> - **Infective endocarditis**
> - **Other conditions** such as cirrhosis of the liver and, to a minor extent, ulcerative colitis, Crohn's disease and occasionally autoimmune thyrotoxicosis
>
> *Note:* Clubbing does *not* occur with chronic obstructive lung disease

Nails

Personal care

This is indicated by observing whether the nails are bitten, painted, clean, dirty and neglected, neatly cut or unusually long.

Splinter haemorrhages

These are small haemorrhages characteristically under the distal part of the nails, as shown in Fig. 4.3. In descending order of frequency, the causes of splinter haemorrhages are:

1. trauma, most commonly as a result of manual work
2. arteritis, that is, inflammation of small arteries
3. infective endocarditis.

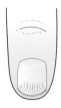

Fig 4.3 Splinter haemorrages

Koilonychia

This is a spoon or concave shape of the nail in its transverse diameter that is occasionally seen with severe iron deficiency.

Pitting

Pitting is pin-sized holes in the nails that are seen in association with psoriasis.

White nails

Statistically, white nails are associated with chronic liver disease, but they also occasionally occur in healthy people.

Yellow nails

Yellow nails are occasionally seen with bronchiectasis.

Anaemia

In the hands, anaemia causes a variable degree of paleness of the nails and palmar surfaces of the fingers, as described on page 33.

Cyanosis and Raynaud's disease/phenomenon

These are described on pages 33 and 41.

Quincke's sign

Quincke's sign is visible pulsation of the capillaries in the pulp of the fingers due to the wide pulse pressure associated with *aortic regurgitation.* It may be demonstrated by placing a lighted torch over a nail and observing it through the tip of the finger. Alternatively, it may also be demonstrated by pressing a glass slide against the lips.

Sweaty palms

The palms are normally dry. Sweaty palms occur with anxiety, thyrotoxicosis or very occasionally a condition of excessive sweating known as hyperhydrosis.

Dupuytren's contracture

Dupuytren's contracture is part of a syndrome of proliferation of fibrous tissue that, in the hand, causes thickening and then contraction of the palmar aponeurosis and its extensions up onto the fingers. It results initially in puckering of the skin of the palm and then in various degrees of flexion deformity of the fourth and fifth fingers that prevents them from being straightened and may interfere with the functions of the hand (Fig. 4.4).

Dupuytren's contracture is associated with:

● increasing age and male sex

● heavy alcohol intake, independently of liver disease

● heavy smoking

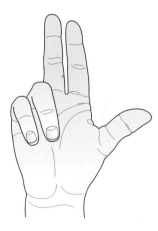

Fig 4.4 Severe Dupuytren's contracture showing fixed flexion of the fourth and fifth fingers

● diabetes mellitus

● possibly manual occupations and epilepsy.

Palmar erythema

Palmar erythema is an abnormal pink/red coloration of the base of the palms that is seen in alcoholic liver disease. It is said to be caused by vasodilatation resulting from failure of the cirrhotic liver to metabolize oestrogens.

Marfan's syndrome

This is a systemic condition that, in the hands, is associated with abnormally long fingers with a ratio of phalangeal bone length to breadth of more than 8:1 or 9:1.

Down's syndrome

This is a systemic condition that, in the hands, is associated with short stubby fingers and a simian crease.

Osler's nodes

Osler's nodes are painful red areas in the pads of the fingers caused by emboli or autoimmune phenomena associated with infective endocarditis.

Pigmentation of the creases of the palm

This is an abnormal brown pigmentation of the palmar creases that applies only to Caucasians, as non-Caucasians have natural pigmentation in the creases of the palm. In Caucasians, palmar pigmentation is a sign of Addison's disease due to *primary adrenal insufficiency*; it results from the increased production of melanocyte-stimulating hormone that accompanies the increased production of adrenocorticotrophic hormone associated with the condition.

Palmar pigmentation *does not* occur with Addison's disease caused by *primary pituitary insufficiency*, as both adrenocorticotrophic hormone and melanocyte-stimulating hormone secretion are depressed and lower than normal in that condition.

Neuropathy

The following may be seen:

- wasting of the thenar eminence due to pathology of the median nerve, most commonly in the carpal tunnel

- wasting of the hypothenar eminence and interosseus muscles due to pathology of the ulnar nerve, most commonly at the elbow.

THE SKIN

The information included in this section is of a general nature. For information about specific conditions of the skin, the student is advised to consult a textbook of dermatology.

> **Box 4.9: General information about lesions of the skin**
>
> - Macule = a flat, non-palpable lesion
> - Papule = an elevated, palpable lesion
> - Nodule = a small lump or knot <1 cm in diameter
> - Plaque = an elevated solid area >1 cm in diameter
> - Wheal = a red, oedematous, inflammatory swelling of the skin, often accompanied by intense itching as part of the reaction to an allergen or irritant
> - Vesicle = a blister < 0.5 cm in diameter
> - Bullous = a blister > 0.5 cm in diameter
> - Breaks in the skin
>   - Erosion = superficial loss of epidermis
>   - Ulcer = deeper loss of skin
>   - Fissure = a linear crack

Specific features of the examination of the skin

During examination of the various systems of the body, note any abnormalities of the skin, such as the following:

- The **character and distribution** of any rashes and whether the skin appears to be of an abnormal texture or is jaundiced or inflamed.

● **Telangiectasia,** that is, small dilated blood vessels. Telangiectasia is a feature of scleroderma and skin that has been irradiated. Spider angiomas (also known as spider naevi) are a specific form of telangiectasis that are described on page 142.

● **Bruises** (bleeds into the skin), that can be classified as:
  ○ **petechiae**: pinpoint haemorrhages, often in association with a low platelet count (thrombocytopenia)

● **purpura**: small haemorrhages, larger than petechiae, that are often seen in association with a low platelet count, vasculitis (inflammation of the walls of small blood vessels) or meningococcal septicaemia
  ○ **echymoses**: bruises or haemorrhages, usually as a result of trauma, a coagulation deficiency or thin-walled leaky blood vessels, such as occur in old age or with prolonged corticosteroid therapy.

Skin tumours

Basal cell carcinoma (rodent ulcer)

This is a tumour that occurs mainly on sun-exposed areas of the face and the back of the hands. Basal cell carcinoma initially presents as a small waxy nodule that slowly develops into an ulcer surrounded by a pearly rolled border, although it may also take other forms. Basal cell carcinomas do not metastasize.

Squamous cell carcinoma

Squamous cell carcinomas are tumours that also occur mainly on sun-exposed areas of the face and hands, where they present as a scaly nodule or mass that often infiltrates locally and has the potential to metastasize.

Malignant melanoma

Malignant melanoma is a highly malignant tumour that should be suspected in any mole of recent onset or an established mole that has undergone change, as about 50 per cent of these tumours, which are derived from melanocytes, originate in moles. The diagnosis is aided by the following 'A, B, C, D' aid to memory:

● A = Asymmetry

● B = Border: an irregular border with local infiltration suggests a melanoma

● C = Colour: the presence of several different colours suggests melanoma

● D = Diameter >6 mm.

Note!

Histologically, the prognosis of patients with malignant melanoma is related to the depth of the lesion.

Kaposi cell sarcoma

This is a highly malignant, red tumour that results from the proliferation of blood vessels in the skin and other parts of the body, most commonly in association with acquired immune deficiency syndrome.

5

VITAL SIGNS

The vital signs

- Temperature
- Radial pulse
- Respiratory rate
- Blood pressure
- Height
- Weight
- Body mass index (BMI)

Equipment needed

- Glass thermometer, or electric thermometer with disposable plastic covers
- Stethoscope
- Sphygmomanometer (blood pressure cuff)
- Watch with a second hand
- Height ruler/scales/BMI chart

Position of the patient

- The patient should be either sitting or lying comfortably in warm, quiet surroundings

EXAMINATION

Taking the temperature

The temperature may be measured at several different sites: orally, rectally, in the axilla or aurally (i.e. via the ear):

● Use an appropriate oral or rectal glass thermometer placed under the tongue or in the rectum or axilla for 2 minutes before reading, or an electric thermometer left to equilibrate under the tongue or in the rectum, axilla or ear before reading.

● Always shake a glass thermometer down before using it. Wash and disinfect the thermometer between patients.

● Always place a disposable plastic cover over an electric thermometer before using it.

● When taking the temperature rectally, ask the patient to lie in the *left lateral position*, that is, on his left side with his knees and hips flexed. Only the tip of the thermometer should be inserted into the rectum.

● When taking the temperature via the axilla, the patient should be asked to adduct his arm tightly against the chest wall once the thermometer has been put in place.

● The normal oral temperature is 37°C (98.6°F).

● The rectal and aural temperatures are about a degree higher than the oral temperature, and the axillary temperature is about a degree lower.

Radial pulse

● Palpate the radial artery, using the tips of at least two or preferably three fingers laid along the length of the artery just above the lateral side of the front of the wrist.

● The three parameters of the pulse that should be monitored are its *rate, rhythm* and *character:*

○ **Pulse rate:** Count the rate for 15 or 30 seconds and multiply by four or two, respectively. The accepted normal rate at rest is between 60 and 100 beats per minute, although in the author's opinion, a rate at rest of over 84 beats per minute is unusually fast.

○ **Pulse rhythm and character:** Determine whether the rhythm is *regular or irregular*, and determine the character, that is, its *amplitude* (size) and *contour* (shape).

Note!

Background information about abnormalities of the rate, rhythm and character of the pulse is on page 60.

Respiratory rate and pattern

● Because breathing is under voluntary control and will unwittingly change if the patient is aware that you are counting his respiratory rate, it is best to count it while still holding the arm and appearing to take the radial pulse.

● The easiest way of counting the respiratory rate is by counting the movements of the chest as the patient breaths in and out for half a minute and then multiplying the result by two. Alternatively, count for a minute. In adults, the rate at rest is normally 14–20 breaths per minute. Rapid breathing is known as *tachypnoea*.

● Apart from counting the respiratory rate, also note the *pattern* of breathing.

Note!

Background information about the respiratory pattern is on page 128.

Blood pressure

- The patient should be sitting at rest on a chair or lying flat in warm, quiet surroundings.

- Choose a cuff of the correct size. The width of the cuff should be approximately 40 per cent of the circumference of the upper arm. Cuffs of the appropriate size are available for normal adults, adults with unusually large arms, children and infants.

- Wrap the cuff round the patient's upper arm so that its lower edge is about 2 cm above the fold in the antecubital fossa.

- Support the patient's arm with your arm or on a bedside table so that the antecubital fossa is at the same level as the patient's heart.

- While you are learning to take the blood pressure, find the approximate *systolic* pressure by *palpating* the pulse at the wrist and noting the pressure at which the pulse disappears as the cuff is inflated. This is the approximate systolic pressure.

- Having determined the approximate systolic pressure, deflate the cuff.

- Now palpate the brachial artery lying slightly medial to the biceps tendon in the antecubital fossa and place the diaphragm of your stethoscope over its pulsation. Inflate the cuff to about 20–30 mmHg above the approximate systolic pressure obtained at the wrist.

- Release the pressure and slowly deflate the cuff at the rate of about 5 mmHg per second.

- The level at which you first hear intermittent beats is the systolic pressure; the sound is due to blood spurting through the artery beneath the cuff and your stethoscope.

- Continue to lower the pressure. The diastolic pressure, which is also known as the Korotkoff phase V, is the pressure at which the sound *disappears* as the flow of blood through the artery becomes continuous and is no longer in spurts. The pressure at which the sounds sometimes *muffle* is known as the Korotkoff phase IV, and is ignored unless the pressure at Korotkoff V is very low, for example 10 mmHg.

● Record both the systolic and diastolic pressures, for example '120/80 mmHg'.

● On the first occasion you take the blood pressure of a particular patient, repeat the reading on the other arm. A difference over 10 mmHg suggests narrowing of an artery in the arm in which the pressure is lower.

Note!

Background information about the blood pressure is on page 68.

Height, weight and height–weight relationship

Height

● Ask the patient to take off his shoes, and then measure his height in centimetres or inches.

Weight

● Measure the patient's weight in kilograms or pounds while he is wearing light clothing without shoes.

Weight–height relationship

● Figure 5.1 shows the relationship between height, weight and state of nutrition and is based on the concept of BMI, which is calculated from the formula BMI = body weight in kg/height in metres^2

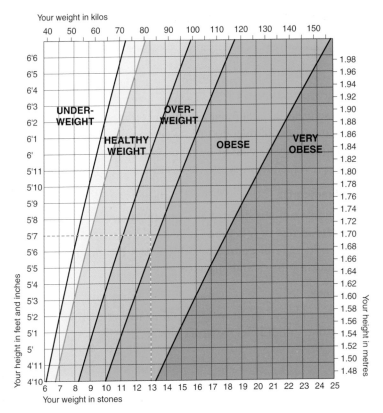

Fig 5.1 Weight–height chart (based on body mass index). Reproduced with permission of the Food Standards Agency

○ Underweight = BMI <18.5
○ Healthy weight = BMI 18.5–24.9
○ Overweight = BMI 25–29.9
○ Obese = BMI 30–34.9
○ Very obese = BMI >35.

BACKGROUND INFORMATION

Rhythm of the pulse

Abnormalities of a regular pulse

Sinus tachycardia

Sinus tachycardia is defined as sinus rhythm with a regular pulse rate at rest of over 100 beats per minute. Sinus tachycardia may be caused by many conditions including anxiety, fever, shock, thyrotoxicosis and rest after exercise.

Sinus bradycardia

Sinus bradycardia is defined as sinus rhythm with a regular pulse rate at rest of less than 60 beats per minute. Sinus bradycardia may be caused by athleticism, hypothyroidism, beta-blocking drugs and jaundice.

Heart block

A regular pulse of about or below 40 beats per minute is usually due to third-degree heart block.

Irregular pulse classified in descending order of frequency

Extrasystoles (ectopic beats)

Ectopic beats or extrasystoles are the most common cause of an irregular pulse and are caused by an ectopic electrical focus in either the atrium or the ventricle firing off at intervals and creating contractions of the heart that interrupt regular sinus rhythm (Fig. 5.2).

Extrasystoles occur early before the next sinus beat and are followed by a gap in the pulse known as a *compensatory pause*, which is due to the refractoriness of the heart muscle following the extrasystole; this prevents the next sinus beat being propagated.

Extrasystoles are usually easy to differentiate, as *they cause irregularities against a background pulse that is basically regular.*

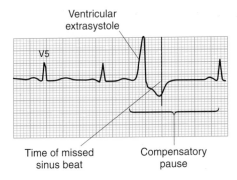

Fig 5.2 Electrocardiograph (ECG) tracing of an extrasytole

Extrasystoles occurring in healthy people are normally of no clinical significance. In the presence of heart disease, however, they may indicate an impaired prognosis.

Atrial fibrillation

Atrial fibrillation is the next most common cause of an irregular pulse and is due to loss of coordinated contraction of the muscle fibres of the atrium, which as a result contract individually in a haphazard, disorganized way. This results in hundreds of electrical impulses arriving in an irregular fashion at the atrioventricular node. However, only a minority of these impulses are greater than the electrical threshold for stimulation of the node. Those that are greater (and are not blocked by the refractory period of the node) pass into the conducting tissue in an irregular manner to stimulate ventricular contractions that are irregular.

Because of this, the pulse of atrial fibrillation is invariably *highly irregular and disorganized with no discernible pattern*. In addition, *the pulse also varies in volume* as the time available for ventricular filling varies between beats. Atrial fibrillation is most commonly caused by myocardial infarction, ischaemic heart disease, hypertensive heart disease, mitral stenosis or regurgitation, and hyperthyroidism.

Irregular heart block

Irregular heart block is the least common cause of an irregular pulse. Atrial flutter is an example of this. In this condition, the atrium contracts regularly at between 230 and 330 beats per minute. In most (but not all) cases, the atrioventricular node is unable to conduct all the electrical impulses associated with such fast contractions of the atrium. This results in a degree of heart block.

If a regular number of impulses are transmitted through the node and into the conducting tissue, the contractions of the ventricle and the pulse are regular. If, on the other hand, the block at the node varies from beat to beat, an irregular number of electrical impulses from the atrium are conducted through the node, and the contractions of the ventricle and the pulse are irregular.

The causes of atrial flutter are similar to the causes of atrial fibrillation.

Character of the pulse

See Box 5.1 and Figure 5.3 for details.

Box 5.1: Character of the pulse: checklist of the more important abnormal pulses

- Atherosclerotic pulse
- Small-volume pulse
- Small-volume, slow-rising pulse
- Bounding pulse
- Waterhammer pulse
- Jerky pulse
- Pulsus alternans
- Pulsus paradoxus
- Pulsus bisferiens

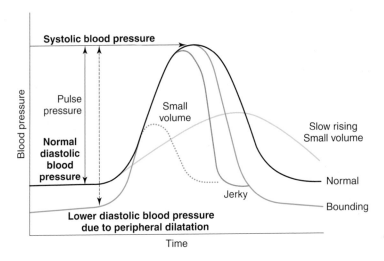

Fig 5.3 Pulses

Atherosclerotic pulse

This can be difficult to elucidate. Palpate the radial pulse and try to determine whether its wall is soft and normal, or hard and atherosclerotic.

Small-volume pulse

A small-volume pulse, which may be weak and difficult to palpate, is found in: severe cardiac failure; low cardiac output shock due, for instance, to a large haemorrhage or myocardial infarction; cardiac tamponade due to pericardial effusion; and massive pulmonary embolus.

Small-volume, slow-rising pulse

A small-volume, slow-rising pulse is an important sign of aortic stenosis. Because the orifice of the aortic valve is narrowed, the rate of ejection of blood from the left ventricle is slow. As a consequence, the volume of the pulse is small and only slowly reaches a maximum.

Large-volume bounding pulse

A large-volume bounding pulse occurs with exercise and is also an important sign in patients suffering from anxiety, anaemia and thyrotoxicosis. What happens is that peripheral dilatation occurs, and as a result there is a slight fall in diastolic pressure, an increase in stroke volume and widening of the pulse pressure (the difference between the systolic and diastolic pressures). These changes are perceived as a large pulse with a *bounding* quality.

Waterhammer pulse

A waterhammer pulse (so-called after a Victorian toy) is a particular type of bounding pulse that is found in aortic regurgitation. It is due to a combination of factors that include peripheral dilatation and blood falling back into the left ventricle during diastole. As a result, this type of pulse is an exaggerated form of a bounding pulse.

The blood falling back into the heart has both systolic and diastolic effects on the pulse. In *diastole*, the volume of blood falling back is added to the blood arriving in the ventricle from the lungs. This leads to an increase in the end-diastolic volume, which in turn leads to an increase in the stroke volume and the width of the pulse pressure during *systole* and an increase in the size of the pulse that is palpated. In addition, the blood falling *back* into the heart also has a *diastolic* effect on the pulse by causing the diastolic pressure to fall further than it would as a result of vasodilatation alone.

The combination of these effects results in a very large widening of the pulse pressure and a strength and character of the pulse that is *best perceived by firmly gripping the forearm between the fingers of your right hand in front and thumb behind*. With the grip maintained and the pulse beneath your fingers just *not* palpable, the patient's forearm is then raised to the level of the head. The occurrence of a thudding pulse under the fingers indicates that the patient has a waterhammer pulse and probably has marked aortic regurgitation.

Jerky pulse

A jerky pulse is a pulse of short duration that is found in mitral regurgitation and hypertrophic cardiomyopathy.

In *mitral regurgitation*, a jerky pulse occurs as a result of blood flowing preferentially back through the incompetent valve into the low-pressure left atrium during systole, rather than into the aorta where the pressure is high. Because the pressure within the left atrium is low, the flow of blood into it from the ventricle is rapid, and as a result ventricular systole is of short duration, producing a pulse that is perceived to be jerky.

In *hypertrophic cardiomyopathy*, a jerky pulse occurs as a result of two main factors. First, the hypertrophied muscle associated with the condition encroaches into the cavity of the left ventricle, reducing stroke volume. Second, hypertrophied muscle in the outflow tract beneath the aortic valve contracts more quickly than the remaining muscle of the ventricle, cutting off the ejection of blood before systole is complete, and so contributes to the perception of a jerky pulse.

Note!

In some respects, hypertrophic cardiomyopathy may be compared with aortic stenosis, as it may produce a somewhat similar triad of symptoms to those listed on page 106.

Pulsus alternans

Pulsus alternans (Fig. 5.4) is an uncommon sign of left ventricular failure characterized by alternating normal and weak beats. The weak beats are caused by the diseased heart muscle failing to recover completely after each normal beat.

Pulsus paradoxus

Pulsus paradoxus (Fig. 5.5) is a *fall of blood pressure during inspiration* and is a common sign in severe asthma, as well as

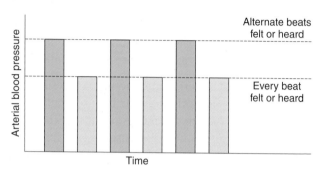

Fig 5.4 Pulsus alternans

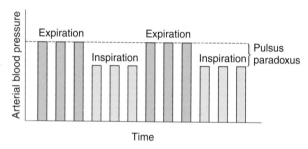

Fig 5.5 Pulsus paradoxus

in constrictive pericarditis, and cardiac tamponade caused by pericardial effusion.

However, pulsus paradoxus is also found to a minor degree in healthy people. What happens in normal health is that, during inspiration, the pressure in the thorax falls, 'sucking out' and increasing the capacity of thin-walled pulmonary vessels such as capillaries and small veins. As a consequence, during inspiration, blood pools in these vessels rather than flowing forward into the heart as it does during expiration when the pressure in the thorax increases and compresses the vessels. The result is a small fall in cardiac output and blood pressure during inspiration.

This phenomenon is greatly exaggerated in asthma. Because the airways are narrowed in asthma, the flow of air into the lungs during inspiration is slow compared with normal. As a result of the slow flow of air into the lungs, the fall in intrathoracic pressure is greater than normal as the lungs expand and their volume increases. This results in greater 'sucking out' of the blood vessels and greater than normal pooling of blood and failure of the blood to flow forward into the heart during inspiration. As a consequence, cardiac output and blood pressure fall even more than normal. Falls greater than 10 mmHg are generally agreed to signify severe asthma.

In cardiac tamponade and constrictive pericarditis, a different mechanism occurs. In addition to the very slight degree of pulsus paradoxus described above in normal people, in these conditions the heart changes shape and tends to hang in the thorax as the patient breathes in. As a result, the pressure exerted by the fluid or tissue constricting the heart increases during inspiration, with the result that even less blood than normal enters the heart, and cardiac output and blood pressure fall more than normally.

Pulsus paradoxus is most easily measured by using a sphygmomanometer and noting the difference in the systolic blood pressure during inspiration compared with expiration.

Pulsus bisferiens

Pulsus bisferiens (Fig. 5.6) is a pulse consisting of two peaks and is a rare sign of aortic regurgitation and hypertrophic cardiomyopathy that is most easily perceived by palpating the brachial or femoral artery. In *aortic regurgitation*, pulsus bisferiens results from blood flowing out from the heart in systole and then flowing back through the incompetent valve in diastole. In *hypertrophic* cardiomyopathy, the first peak is due to ventricular systole, and the second peak or 'tidal wave' is due to blood flowing back to the centre from the periphery as a result of systole stopping suddenly as the outflow tract from the heart closes before ventricular systole is over.

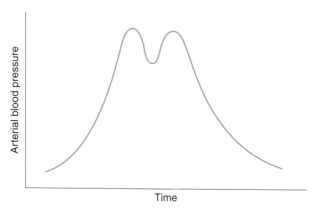

Fig 5.6 Pulsus bisferiens

Blood pressure

The blood pressure depends upon cardiac output and peripheral resistance.

● **Systolic pressure** depends upon cardiac output and the resistance to its ejection into the arterial tree.

● **Diastolic pressure** is the pressure in the arterial tree when the aortic valve is closed and there is no pumping action of the heart. Diastolic pressure is dependent upon the elasticity in the walls of the arteries exerting pressure and 'squeezing' the blood forward during diastole.

Hypertension is somewhat arbitrarily defined as a sustained systolic and/or a diastolic pressure of over 140/90 mmHg, measured on several occasions in a relaxed patient.

6

HEAD, NOSE, MOUTH, EARS AND NECK

Equipment needed

- Spatula or tongue depressor
- Bright light for inspecting the mouth (this may be from either an otoscope or a torch)
- Otoscope fitted with the largest speculum
- Glass of water

Position of the patient

- The patient should be sitting comfortably in warm, quiet surroundings
- Remember to ask the patient before palpating or probing any of the structures involved in these examinations

---

EXAMINATION

Head

Inspection and palpation

Face

- Inspect the face, noting its shape and symmetry, the patient's mood, non-verbal communication, involuntary movements, any swelling, including swelling of the parotid gland, arcus senilis, cyanosis, anaemia, basal and squamous cell carcinomas or any of the signs listed in Chapter 4.

Hair

● Use your fingers or a spatula to part the hair and inspect its distribution, noting its texture, for example whether it is coarse as in hypothyroidism or fine as in hyperthyroidism, and whether there are any lice, nits or alopecia.

Scalp

● Inspect and palpate the scalp for masses, scars, ulcers, the scaliness of psoriasis, dandruff or seborrhoeic dermatitis (which is dandruff associated with inflammation of the scalp) and, if appropriate, the tenderness of temporal arteritis.

Skull

● Inspect and palpate the bones of the skull, noting their shape and any asymmetry, tenderness, masses or enlargement of the head or parts of the head due to hydrocephalus or Paget's disease of bone.

Nose

Inspection

● Look for deviation and any deformities.

Palpation

● Test for tenderness by gently lifting the tip of the nose with your index finger and also by gently squeezing the bridge of the nose between your thumb and index finger.

● Test for nasal obstruction by occluding one nostril at a time and asking the patient to breathe through the other.

● Test for tenderness over the frontal and maxillary sinuses by pressing gently with the tips of your thumbs. Tenderness suggests inflammation of the sinuses, that is, sinusitis.

Inspection of the inside of the nose

● Fit the largest speculum to an otoscope and hold the instrument in your right hand to inspect the left side of the nose, so that its handle points laterally and you are able to steady it by placing your little finger on the patient's cheek.

● Gently insert the speculum about 1 cm into the entrance of the nose, taking care to avoid contact with the sensitive nasal mucosa, and then carefully inspect the septum, looking for deviation, perforation or ulcers suggesting use of cocaine.

● Inspect the mucosa on both the septum and lateral sides of the nose looking for signs of inflammation (purple with allergy, red with infection).

● Inspect the turbinates on the lateral side of the nose, and look superiorly for polyps, which are smooth and often look like a grape and are frequently seen in association with allergy.

● Repeat the examination on the other side of the nose using your left hand to hold the instrument.

Mouth

● If necessary, ask the patient to remove any lipstick or dentures.

● Use a spatula or tongue depressor to aid you as necessary.

Inspection

A list of the structures to be inspected is contained in the checklist box on page 72.

> ✔ **checklist of structures to be inspected in the mouth**
>
> - Lips
> - Buccal mucosa
> - Tongue
> - Floor of the mouth
> - Teeth and gums
> - Hard palate
> - Soft palate, including movements of the uvula
> - Anterior and posterior tonsillar pillars
> - Tonsils or tonsillar bed
> - Pharynx

- At each site, look for ulcers, tumours, leukoplakia (white patches of hyperkeratosis of the squamous epithelium that will not rub away and are sometimes precancerous), and signs of infection, such as inflammation of the tonsils, inflammation of the back of the soft palate suggestive of herpangina or generalized small white patches suggestive of monilia. A high-arch palate is seen in Marfan's syndrome.

Particular aspects of the examination of the mouth

Lips

- Look at the lips for the blueness of cyanosis or the pallor of anaemia, and at the angles of the mouth for angular cheilitis, which is fissuring of the angles seen with deficiency of:
  - ○ vitamin B_2 (riboflavin)
  - ○ vitamin B_6 (pyridoxine)
  - ○ iron.

Tongue

- **Movements of the tongue:** ask the patient to protrude his tongue and observe its surface and the way it moves. Abnormalities of its movement are discussed on page 189.

- Colour and surface of the tongue:
  - ○ A *pale, smooth tongue* with an *atrophic* epithelium is seen in iron-deficiency anaemia.
  - ○ A *red smooth tongue* is seen in deficiencies of vitamins B_2, B_6 and B_{12}.
  - ○ A *bright red tongue* is seen in pellagra owing to a deficiency of vitamin B_3 (niacin).
  - ○ A *white fury tongue* is seen in moniliasis associated with antibiotic therapy.

Note!

The tongue of many healthy people has a putty-coloured coating that is of no clinical significance.

Gums and teeth

- Look at the state of dental hygiene and whether or not the teeth and gums are healthy.

Movement of the uvula

This is a test of cranial nerves IX and X, both of which supply motor fibres to the pharynx.

- Ask the patient to open his mouth and say 'Ah' as you watch his uvula. If necessary, use a light to illuminate the mouth. Movement of the uvula is normally symmetrically upwards, or *away from* the side of any weakness, as the muscles on the normal side contract and pull the uvula towards them. Weakness may result in slurred speech known as *dysarthria*, which is discussed on page 192.

Malfunction of cranial nerves IX and X may be caused by:

- strokes
- pharyngeal cancer invading the nerves
- motor neurone disease.

Sensation of the pharynx

This is a test of the sensory component of cranial nerves IX and X, both of which supply sensory fibres to the pharynx.

● Inform the patient about what you intend to do and, if he agrees, ask him to open his mouth wide. Now evoke the gag reflex by touching the back of his pharynx with a tongue depressor or Q-tip. Failure to gag suggests either sensory or motor loss to the pharynx.

Ears

Inspection

● Inspect the pinna for deformities, inflammation, scars, tumours or lumps such as gouty tophi, which consist of hard deposits of sodium urate crystals around the periphery of the pinna.

Palpation

● Gently press on the tragus (the small triangular structure at the front of the ear). Pain suggests otitis externa (inflammation of the external auditory canal).

● Gently press on the mastoid bones on either side behind the ears. Pain or tenderness suggests inflammation (mastoiditis).

Otoscopic examination

● Fit the otoscope with the largest speculum that will fit comfortably into the ear.

● Pull the ear gently backwards and upwards to straighten the auditory canal, and gently insert the speculum about 1 cm into the canal, using the same technique as you did for the nose.

● Then, *keeping your eye, the line of light, the orifices of the instrument and the line of the auditory canal in one straight line,* inspect the canal, looking for wax or for inflammation indicating otitis externa.

● Finally, inspect the eardrum, which is normally greyish-black and shiny due to the light shining back into your eye. Note the malleus and look for any redness, bulging or inflammation of the tympanic membrane suggestive of otitis media, any perforations, or a fluid level indicating serous effusion.

Hearing tests

These are usually performed as part of the examination of cranial nerve VIII and are discussed on page 172.

Neck

Inspection

● Look for asymmetry, masses, scars or enlargement of the thyroid gland, salivary glands or lymph nodes. Also look to see whether the trachea appears to be central or deviated to one side.

Palpation

Lymph nodes

Palpate both sides simultaneously with the fingertips of both your hands as follows and as illustrated in Fig. 6.1, noting any enlargement or tenderness of the:

● buccal nodes – posterior to the lips

● superficial parotid nodes – anterior to the inferior angle of the pinna of the ear

● postauricular nodes – adjacent to the mastoid bone behind the ear

● occipital nodes – adjacent to the occipital protuberance

● tonsillar nodes – in the neck immediately beneath the angle of the jaw

● submandibular and submental nodes – beneath the mandible

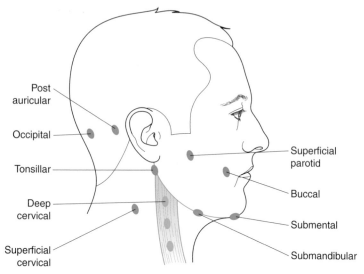

Fig 6.1 Lymph nodes of the head and neck

- two chains of cervical nodes:
  - ○ superficial – posterior to the sternomastoid muscle
  - ○ deep – deep to the sternomastoid muscle, along the internal jugular vein

- supraclavicular nodes – lateral to the sternomastoid muscle and immediately above the medial end of the clavicle.

> ### Note!
>
> Small shotty glands may be felt in healthy people. Pain and tenderness suggest infection. Hard irregular enlargement that is deeply attached suggests metastases from a carcinoma, for example thyroid, nasopharyngeal or bronchus. Rubbery enlargement suggests lymphoma.

Trachea

- Ask the patient to look straight ahead, and then inspect to see whether the trachea appears to be central or deviated to one side.

- Palpate the trachea by one or both of the following methods to determine whether or not it is central:
  - ○ Run a single finger down the centre of the trachea and determine whether it runs through the centre of the suprasternal notch or whether it is deviated to one side.
  - ○ Run each of your index fingers, or the index and middle fingers of your right hand, down either side of the trachea and determine whether it is central or deviated to one side by referring to the medial ends of the clavicles.

- The causes of deviation of the trachea are discussed on page 129.

Thyroid gland

- From the **front**:
  - ○ Palpate the gland from the front by simultaneously running the middle and index fingers of each of your hands down either side of the trachea from the level of the larynx. Alternatively, place the index and middle fingers of your right hand on either side of the trachea at the level of the larynx and run them down either side of the trachea.
  - ○ The gland is usually barely palpable. If it is palpable, note its size and whether it is diffusely enlarged, enlarged on one side or nodular.

- From **behind**: now go behind the patient and:
  - ○ place the index and middle fingers of both your hands over the cricoid cartilage just beneath the level of the larynx
  - ○ ask the patient to take a mouthful of water and hold it in his mouth
  - ○ now ask him to swallow the water while you note whether the gland rises and slides up under your fingers
  - ○ note any palpable abnormalities of the gland.

BACKGROUND INFORMATION

Goitres

A goitre is a visible/palpable swelling of the thyroid gland. The main questions to be answered about a goitre are:

- Is the patient hyperthyroid or euthyroid/hypothyroid?

- Is the goitre diffuse or nodular?

With this information, it is an easy matter to select the appropriate group of diagnoses (Fig. 6.2). Remember, however, that only approximately 50 per cent of patients with hyperthyroidism have a goitre. The other 50 per cent have either an impalpable nodule or a diffusely overactive gland without any visible or palpable swelling.

Autoimmune hypothyroidism (Hashimoto's disease) is often associated with a goitre; primary hypothyroidism, the cause of which is unknown (although it may be a burnt-out form of Hashimoto's disease), is not usually associated with a goitre.

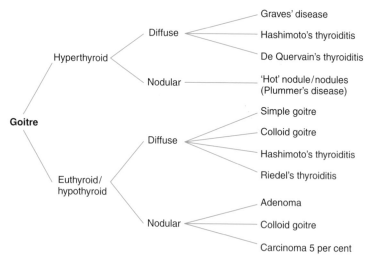

Fig 6.2 Classification of goitre

Nodules associated with euthyroidism and hypothyroidism are important because about 5 per cent are due to carcinoma. Because of this, all such nodules of recent or fairly recent onset must be biopsied.

7

CARDIOVASCULAR SYSTEM

Equipment needed
- Stethoscope
- Sphygmomanometer
- Bright light
- Ruler and straight edge

Position of the patient
- The patient should be covered and lying comfortably in warm, quiet surroundings with his trunk and head elevated at an angle of about 30–45°
- It is suggested that you follow the order of the examination in this chapter, as it is typical of the order used in clinical practice and will help you not to forget anything. Start by inspecting the face and the patient generally, then move to the hands, and then move proximally up the right arm to the radial pulse, the neck and finally the precordium and heart.

Order of the examination
- Inspection
- Palpation
- Percussion
- Auscultation

EXAMINATION

General inspection and inspection of the face (relevant to the cardiovascular system)

- Inspect the face and upper part of the body, noting any breathlessness, use of accessory muscles, central cyanosis, anaemia, arcus senilis or xanthomata.

Inspection of the hands (relevant to the cardiovascular system)

- Look for cyanosis, clubbing of the fingers, splinter haemorrhages and Osler's nodes

Examination of the radial pulse

- If you have not already done so as part of the vital signs, palpate the radial artery, using the tips of at least two or preferably three fingers laid along the length of the artery just above the wrist.

- The three parameters of the radial pulse that should be monitored are its *rate*, *rhythm* and *character*.

- A full description of these parameters is discussed on pages 56 and 60.

Examination of the neck

Carotid artery

Inspection

- Inspect the right side of the neck, looking for any visible pulsation.

- A bright light positioned to shine either directly or tangentially onto the neck may be helpful.

- If necessary, ask the patient if you may move his head. Do this by placing your index and middle fingers under the patient's chin and gently lifting and turning his head to the left until you have an optimal view of any pulsation in the neck.

- If a pulsation is visible, it is important to determine whether it is from the carotid artery or the internal jugular vein.

- The way to distinguish between the two is to appreciate that pulsation from the carotid artery is most commonly seen under the angle of the jaw and consists of a *single* pulsation, whereas, as explained below, the level of any pulsation from the internal jugular vein varies and, if the patient is in sinus rhythm, consists of *three* pulsations.

Palpation

- Palpate with your thumb or the tips of two or three fingers beneath the angle of the jaw to determine the character of the pulse in the carotid artery (the most important findings are discussed in the Note below).

Auscultation

- Auscultate for bruits over both carotid arteries with the diaphragm of your stethoscope.

- Bruits are harsh continuous *Ssssh* or *Crrrh* systolic sounds that sound like systolic murmurs, and are due to the turbulence created by blood flowing out from a narrowing in an artery, in this case the carotid artery.

Note!

A similar sound over the carotid artery may be due to radiation of the systolic murmur of aortic stenosis.

Also note that the carotid artery is probably the best site to palpate the small-volume, slow-rising pulse of aortic stenosis, the bounding pulse of aortic regurgitation (known in the neck as *Corrigan's sign*), and the jerky pulse associated with hypertrophic cardiomyopathy and mitral regurgitation.

A description of all these pulses is on pages 62 and 68.

Jugular venous pulse

The jugular venous pulse (JVP; Fig. 7.1) is most commonly used to assess the presence of right heart failure. Measuring it can be difficult. If necessary, use a bright light and position the patient's head as described for the carotid artery.

● Assess the height of the JVP by placing a ruler vertically on the manubriosternal angle (Fig. 7.2), to measure the distance *to the top of the pulsating column of blood* in the internal jugular vein.

● Normally the reading is less than 3 cm. A greater reading indicates right heart failure (or rarely pericardial tamponade or constriction).

● Never use the *external* jugular vein to measure the JVP, as it can be partially occluded by fascial planes in the neck, resulting in a falsely high reading. For a similar reason, never use the *left* internal jugular vein, as it may be compressed in the thorax by the left subclavian artery.

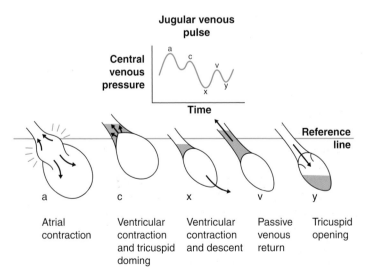

Fig 7.1 Jugular venous pulse

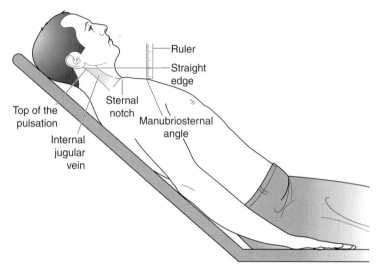

Ruler

Straight edge

Sternal notch

Manubriosternal angle

Top of the pulsation

Internal jugular vein

Fig 7.2 Measuring the JVP

> **Note!**
>
> Background information about the JVP is on page 93.

Box 7.1 outlines the clinical features seen in cardiac failure.

> **Box 7.1: Clinical features of cardiac failure**
>
> **Symptoms**
> - Breathlessness on exertion (dyspnoea) and lying flat (orthopnoea) ± at night (nocturnal dyspnoea)
> - Fatigue, loss of appetite
> - Reduced exercise tolerance
> - Ascending swelling (oedema) of the dependent parts of the body
> - Pain and tenderness in the right upper quadrant of the abdomen due to congestion of the liver

- Nocturia due to oedema moving into the vascular compartment and reduced renovascular constriction on lying recumbent

Signs
- Sometimes none (diagnosis made on the basis of a history of breathless plus investigations)
- Dyspnoea and tachypnoea
- Central cyanosis
- Peripheral oedema
- Signs listed in Table 7.1 (page 110)

Precordium and heart

Inspection

- Look for any movement of the sternal or apical areas. If visible, the apex is just medial to and beneath the nipple in a healthy man.

- Movement of the sternum is a sign of right ventricular hypertrophy.

- Movement of the apex may be seen normally in slim persons but is also a sign of an abnormally powerful heart beat due to left ventricular hypertrophy.

Palpation

The order in which this is usually done, which may be reversed if you wish, is related to the anatomical positions of the important cardiac structures in the chest, and is:

1. second right intercostal space (2RICS), which is immediately inferior to the right side of the manubriosternal angle (the palpable angle or ridge between the manubrium and the sternum)
2. second left intercostal space (2LICS), which is immediately inferior to the left side of the manubriosternal angle
3. lower left sternal edge (LSE)
4. apex.

Details of how to palpate these areas is discussed in the following paragraphs.

2RICS

This is downstream from the aortic valve. Therefore palpate here for palpable information about that valve.

- To do this, place the distal pads of the first three fingers of your right hand flat over the 2RICS and feel for:
  - an aortic component of the second heart sound
  - the vibration of a thrill from the aortic valve.

> **Note!**
>
> Background information about these signs is on pages 93–102.

2LICS

This is downstream from the pulmonary valve and so gives information about that valve.

- Place the distal pads of the first three fingers of your right hand flat over the 2LICS and feel for:
  - a pulmonary component of the second heart sound
  - the vibration of a thrill from the pulmonary valve.

> **Note!**
>
> Background information about these signs is on pages 93–102.

Sternum

- To palpate the sternum, place your right hand flat along its length, slightly to the left of its centre. Alternatively, place the *heel* of your hand along the sternum with the fingers raised and pointing laterally. The latter technique will cause your fingers to act as a lever and will magnify any movement, making it easy to both see and feel any movement.

● At the same time, feel for the vibration of a thrill caused by the murmur of aortic regurgitation or a ventricular septal defect (VSD), or very rarely a lesion of the tricuspid valve. Details of these are discussed on page 105.

Note!

Normally, the sternum does not move. Palpable movement of the sternum is known as a *sternal heave* and is abnormal and usually due to an abnormally powerful right ventricle, that is, right ventricular hypertrophy, although it may very occasionally be due to a *hyperdynamic* right ventricle caused by the increased flow of blood through the pulmonary circulation associated with an atrial septal defect.

Cardiac apex

● To palpate the cardiac apex, place the fingers of your right hand *flat* and pointing laterally across the patient's chest at approximately the intersection of the fifth intercostal space and the mid-clavicular line, that is, just medial to and beneath the nipple in a healthy man.

● If the apex is not palpable in that area, palpate for it laterally in the mid- or even the posterior axillary line.

● If you identify a pulsation, determine its position precisely with the tips of your fingers and note its character.

Note!

Background information about abnormalities of the character of the cardiac apex is on page 93.

If it is palpable, the position of the cardiac apex is described in terms of two parameters:

1. the rib space it occupies
2. a vertical line dropped down from the clavicle or, if appropriate, the anterior, mid- or posterior axillary line.

Determining the position of the cardiac apex in terms of the *rib spaces* can be difficult, particularly in people with an obese or muscular chest wall.

● The way it is done is by counting down the rib spaces along the left sternal edge with the tips of the fingers of your right hand, starting from the 2LICS, which is immediately inferior to the left side of the manubriosternal angle. When you have counted down to the space in which you think the apex is palpable, its position is confirmed by sliding your finger along the space until it is over the pulsation.

To describe the position of the cardiac apex in terms of the *clavicle or axillary lines*:

● The position of the apex is determined relative to the clavicle or axillary lines by dropping an imaginary line vertically down the front or side of the chest to the pulsation you have identified.

Percussion of the heart

Percussion is another method of assessing the size of the heart, and is particularly helpful in cases of cardiac tamponade but is often not accurate enough to be helpful in other cases.

● The technique of percussing the heart is the same as the technique of percussing the chest and is described on page 123.

● In the case of the heart, start in the left mid-axillary line at approximately the level of the fifth intercostal space and percuss horizontally towards the centre, seeking any dullness indicating the left border of the heart. On the right side, start at roughly the same level, or a little higher to avoid hepatic dullness, and percuss horizontally towards the centre of the chest to identify any dullness indicating the right border of the heart.

Auscultation of the heart

> **Note!**
>
> Background information about the various heart sounds and murmurs mentioned in this section is on pages 95–109.

Using a stethoscope correctly

The diaphragm of the stethoscope is designed for listening to high-pitch sounds and the bell for listening to low-pitch sounds. Listen with the diaphragm in all areas, as most heart sounds and murmurs are high pitch. In addition, listen with the bell for the low-pitch rumble of mitral stenosis and the low-pitch sound of the third and fourth heart sounds.

Where to listen

This is related to the anatomical positions of the various valves and is described below. It is suggested that you listen in the following order, which may be reversed if you wish.

First listen in *2RICS*.

- This is downstream from the aortic valve. Therefore listen here for sounds from the aortic valve, namely:
  - ○ loudness or softness of the aortic component of the second heart sound (A_2)
  - ○ murmurs from the aortic valve (stenosis or regurgitation).

Next listen in *2LICS*.

- This is downstream from the pulmonary valve. Therefore listen here for sounds from the pulmonary valve, namely:
  - ○ loudness or softness of the pulmonary component of the second heart sound (P_2) and splitting of the second heart sound (A_2P_2)
  - ○ murmurs from the pulmonary valve (stenosis or regurgitation) or occasionally the flow murmur of an atrial septal defect.

Next, listen at the *lower left sternal edge.*

● This is over the interventricular septum and tricuspid valve, and is also over the direction of the flow of blood back into the heart in aortic regurgitation and pulmonary regurgitation. Therefore listen here for *all* of the following:
  ○ the tricuspid component of the first heart sound
  ○ the murmur of *aortic regurgitation* or rarely the similar-sounding murmur of *pulmonary regurgitation*
  ○ the murmur of a VSD
  ○ murmurs from the tricuspid valve (very rare).

Then listen at the *cardiac apex.*

● The mitral valve is heard best at the cardiac apex. Therefore listen here for sounds from the mitral valve, namely:
  ○ the mitral component of the first heart sound
  ○ murmurs from the mitral valve (regurgitation or stenosis), remembering that the latter is heard best with the bell of the stethoscope.

Next listen *between the apex and left sternal edge.*

● Listen here for the third and fourth heart sounds, remembering to use the bell of the stethoscope.

Finally, perform *two specific manoeuvres* intended to bring the heart closer to the chest wall and the stethoscope:

● Ask the patient to turn onto his left side, exhale and hold his breath while you place the bell of your stethoscope *very lightly* against his cardiac apex and listen for the murmur of mitral stenosis, which may be too soft to hear when the patient is lying on his back.

● Ask the patient to sit up, lean forward and exhale and hold his breath while you listen at the left sternal edge with the diaphragm of the stethoscope for the murmur of aortic regurgitation (or rarely pulmonary regurgitation), which may be too soft to hear when the patient is lying on his back

Completing the examination of the cardiovascular system

If you are examining only the cardiovascular system and not the other systems of the body, complete the examination by performing the following.

Lung bases

● Auscultate the lung bases at the back of the chest for crackles resulting from congestion caused, for instance, by left heart failure. A description of crackles is on page 132.

Lower legs

● Inspect for swelling indicating oedema and, if any is present or suspected, palpate by pressing with your thumb or fingers for at least 5 seconds over the dorsums of the feet, behind the medial malleoli and over the shins. Note any visible indentation. The causes of oedema of the legs are listed on page 107.

Blood pressure

● The final part of the examination of the cardiovascular system is to take the blood pressure, if you have not already taken it as part of the vital signs, as the patient is most likely to be relaxed at this point of the examination.

Table 7.1 summarises information on the cardiac signs.

BACKGROUND INFORMATION

JVP

In right heart failure, a column of blood accumulates in the great veins behind the failing ventricle and becomes visible and therefore measurable in the neck.

Apart from measuring the height of the JVP, it is also possible to analyse the pulsations within it. These are transmitted from the heart, as there is no valve between the right atrium and the superior vena cava to block their transmission.

The JVP normally consists of three pulsations: the 'a' wave, due to atrial contraction sending a spurt of blood back into the venous system; the 'c' wave, due to upward doming of the tricuspid valve into the right atrium during ventricular contraction; and the 'v' wave, due to venous return passively filling the great veins at the end of systole, resulting in an increasing column of blood collecting in the jugular vein. Details of the three waves in the JVP are illustrated in Fig. 7.1 (page 83).

In atrial fibrillation, the 'a' wave is absent and there are only two waves in the JVP.

Abnormally large waves in the JVP

Abnormally large waves in the JVP may occur as a result of blood flowing backwards into the great veins and jugular vein as follows.

Large 'a' (atrial) wave

This is due to:

- **tricuspid stenosis,** resulting in the right atrium contracting against increased resistance and so causing blood to flow backwards into the great veins

- **aortic stenosis,** due to severe left ventricular hypertrophy causing the left ventricle to bulge into the right ventricle and so obstruct the flow of blood through the right side of the heart.

Cannon waves

These are due to:

- **complete heart block or ventricular tachycardia,** resulting in the atria and the ventricles contracting at different rates. As a consequence, the right atrium at times contracts when the tricuspid valve is closed, with the result that blood flows backwards into the great veins.

Large 'v' wave

This is due to:

● **tricuspid regurgitation**, resulting in blood regurgitating backwards through the open valve during right ventricular systole.

Other abnormalities of the JVP

Superior vena cava syndrome

This syndrome presents in the JVP as *non-pulsatile distension of the internal and external jugular veins* due to obstruction of the superior vena cava, most commonly by a constricting bronchial carcinoma.

Venous paradoxus (Kussmaul's sign)

This is a *paradoxical increase in the JVP, causing the neck to become visibly distended during inspiration*, whereas normally, as explained on page 66, the pressure *falls* in the jugular vein as blood is sucked into the thorax during inspiration.

Venous paradoxus is seen in pericardial constriction and tamponade, and is due to the heart changing shape as it descends and 'hangs' in the thorax during inspiration. As a result, the pressure increases in the fluid that has collected around the heart in the pericardial sac, causing it to obstruct the flow of blood from the great veins into the heart.

Cardiac apex

The apical impulse is due to the heart rotating and striking the anterior chest wall as it contracts during systole.

If palpable, the cardiac apex has several components, namely, its *position*, *amplitude*, *character* and *duration*, each of which is discussed in the following paragraphs.

Position of the cardiac apex

Position in health

In health, the cardiac apex is usually not palpable, although it may be in slim persons, in which case it is normally in the fourth or fifth intercostal space, at or inside the mid-clavicular line.

Position in diseased states

Cardiac dilatation may result in the cardiac apex being displaced laterally to the anterior axillary line or even the mid- or posterior axillary line.

> ### Note!
>
> Cardiac dilatation is typically caused by a ventricle failing and being unable to pump out all the blood it receives. As a result, the pressure in the veins filling the ventricle (preload) increases, and the ventricle blows up like a balloon.

Amplitude, character and duration of the cardiac apex

Normal apex

Normally, as stated above, the cardiac apex is either impalpable or a small pulsation of short duration.

Sustained cardiac apex

A sustained cardiac apex is one in which the outer movement of the cardiac impulse takes longer than normal and does not fall away as quickly as normal. A sustained apex is usually the result of *hypertrophy* of the heart muscle.

> ### Note!
>
> *Hypertrophy of cardiac muscle.* Like any other muscle, cardiac muscle grows bigger and stronger and hypertrophies when it continually contracts against increased resistance (afterload), as occurs with hypertension and aortic stenosis. In the absence of dilatation, hypertrophy alone usually results in a sustained apex that is either in the normal position or only a little displaced.

Hyperdynamic cardiac apex

A hyperdynamic cardiac apex is one that is exaggerated due to the outer movement of the cardiac impulse being quicker and larger and falling away more quickly than normal. A hyperdynamic cardiac apex typically occurs in states associated with increased cardiac output, such as exercise, anxiety, thyrotoxicosis and aortic regurgitation.

Double cardiac apex

Conditions occasionally associated with a double cardiac apex are *cardiac aneurysm, aortic stenosis* and *hypertrophic cardiomyopathy*. With a cardiac aneurysm, one pulsation is the normal one and the other is expansion of the aneurysm during systole. With aortic stenosis and hypertrophic cardiomyopathy, the left ventricle becomes very thick and hypertrophied, and in response the left atrium hypertrophies as it endeavours to push blood forward. This results in an unusually powerful left atrium, the contraction of which causes a palpable presystolic filling bulge of the ventricle before the left ventricular thrust.

Tapping apex

As explained on page 98, the first heart sound in mitral stenosis may be so loud as to produce a palpable tap.

Auscultation

Heart sounds

The cardiac cycle normally consists of two heart sounds: the first heart sound and the second heart sound. In heart disease, there may be a third heart sound and/or a fourth heart sound. A systolic click may also be heard.

First heart sound (S_1)

The first heart sound arises from both the mitral and the tricuspid valves and is created by the cusps of the valves striking one another as they close at the beginning of ventricular systole.

Second heart sound (S₂)

The second heart sound is due to both the aortic and pulmonary valves, and is created by the cusps of the valves striking one another as they close at the beginning of ventricular diastole.

Intensity of the heart sounds

The intensity (i.e. loudness/softness) of the first and second heart sounds is due to the *speed* rather than the force with which the cusps of a valve strike one another. As illustrated in Fig. 7.3, on auscultation the first heart sound sounds like *lub* and the second heart sound sounds like *dub*.

Third heart sound (S₃)

The third heart sound is an *audible creak*, usually caused by the expansion of a diseased stiff ventricle at the height of maximal filling during the middle of diastole. A third heart sound is heard in myocardial infarction, heart failure, mitral regurgitation and chronic constrictive pericarditis, and is normal in fit young people under the age of 40 with very rapid filling of the heart.

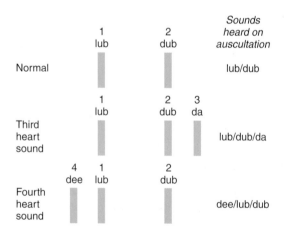

Fig 7.3 Heart sounds

As shown in Fig. 7.3, on auscultation the third heart sound comes after the second heart sound in the middle of diastole, and in relation to the first and second heart sounds, sounds like *lub, dub, da.*

Fourth heart sound (S$_4$)

The fourth heart sound is an *audible ventricular creak* that occurs as the atrium contracts during atrial systole and squeezes a last drop of blood into an already almost filled diseased stiff ventricle, causing it to expand further. A fourth heart sound is always pathological and is heard most commonly in myocardial infarction, hypertension and heart failure.

The symptoms and signs of myocardial infarction are listed in Box 7.2.

Box 7.2: Symptoms and signs of myocardial infarction

Symptoms
- Tight, heavy, constricting or indigestion-like central chest pain at rest or persisting after exertion, often radiating to one or both arms ± the jaw
- Sudden unwellness with sweating, usually with the above type of pain
- Sudden breathlessness due to left ventricular failure
- Sudden unconsciousness due to cardiac arrhythmia

Signs
- None, except possibly a fourth heart sound, *or*:
- Unwell appearance with pallor and sweating due to activation of the sympathetic nervous system
- Sinus rhythm or an arrhythmia, e.g. extrasystoles, sinus bradycardia, sinus tachycardia, atrial fibrillation, atrial flutter, ventricular tachycardia, ventricular fibrillation or first-, second- or third-degree heart block
- Fourth heart sound
- Signs of left ventricular failure (Table 7.1 on page 110)

- New-onset murmur of mitral regurgitation or ventricular septal defect due to rupture of the chordae tendineae or ventricular septum
- Cardiogenic shock, i.e. extreme unwellness and cold sweat with sinus tachycardia, weak pulse, low blood pressure and poor perfusion of the tissues

As shown in Fig. 7.3, a fourth heart sound occurs immediately before the first heart sound, and, in relation to the first and second heart sounds, sounds like *dee, lub, dub.*

Loud heart sounds

Loud first heart sound

The mitral valve normally closes at a moderate speed at the beginning of ventricular systole. In mitral stenosis, however, the valve is stiff and takes longer to close than normal, and when it does so, it is under the full force of ventricular systole. This causes the valve to slam shut very quickly and results in an abnormally loud first heart sound at the apex that may be so pronounced as to be a palpable tap. *An abnormally loud first heart sound at the apex is therefore suggestive of mitral stenosis.*

Loud aortic component of the second heart sound (A₂)

In systemic hypertension, the increased systemic arterial pressure causes the aortic valve to slam shut abnormally quickly, and as a result *in systemic hypertension the second heart sound is usually abnormally loud in the vicinity of the aortic valve (the aortic area), that is, 2RICS.*

Loud pulmonary component of the second heart sound (P₂)

In pulmonary hypertension, the increased pressure in the pulmonary artery causes the pulmonary valve to slam shut abnormally quickly, and as a result *in pulmonary hypertension the second heart sound is usually abnormally loud in the vicinity of the pulmonary valve (the pulmonary area), that is, 2LICS.*

Soft heart sounds

Soft first heart sound

The first heart sound is abnormally soft at the cardiac apex in mitral stenosis when the mitral valve is so stiff that it cannot close properly. Thus, in mitral stenosis, the first heart sound may be either abnormally loud, as described earlier, or abnormally soft (i.e. quiet), as described here.

Soft second heart sound (A$_2$)

The second heart sound is usually abnormally soft in the aortic area (2RICS) in aortic stenosis as the aortic valve is stiff and does not close properly. Thus, all that is usually heard in aortic stenosis is a single component transmitted from the nearby pulmonary valve.

Soft second heart sound (P$_2$)

The second heart sound is usually abnormally soft in the pulmonary area (2LICS) in pulmonary stenosis as the pulmonary valve is stiff and does not close properly. Thus, all that is usually heard in pulmonary stenosis is a single component transmitted from the nearby aortic valve.

Both heart sounds soft

Both heart sounds are usually soft in conditions in which the transmission of sound from the heart to the stethoscope is reduced, as follows:

- a muscular chest wall

- obesity

- cardiac tamponade, due to fluid around the heart

- emphysema, due to the increased volume of lung between the heart and the stethoscope

- immediately after myocardial infarction. In this situation, the heart sounds are said to be *muffled* as a result of poor cardiac contraction.

Splitting of the second heart sound

Physiological splitting of the second heart sound

This is an audible splitting of the second heart sound into two components that occurs in healthy people during inspiration and is explained as follows and is illustrated in Fig. 7.4:

● *During expiration*, the two components of the second heart sound (aortic and pulmonary, i.e. A_2 and P_2) occur together and are heard as one.

● *During inspiration*, the intrathoracic pressure falls, sucking extra blood into the great veins and right side of the heart. As a result, right ventricular systole takes longer than left ventricular systole, so the pulmonary valve closes after the aortic valve, causing a delay in the pulmonary component of the second heart sound.

Fixed splitting of the second heart sound

This is an audible split in the second heart sound into two components *during both inspiration and expiration*, and is explained as follows and as illustrated in Fig. 7.4.

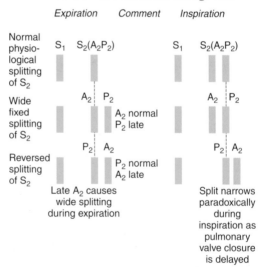

Fig 7.4 Splitting of the second heart sound

With a left-to-right shunt caused by an atrial septal defect, the flow of blood through the lungs and right side heart may be as much as three or four times the flow of blood through left ventricle and out through the aorta. This is because most of the blood returning to the left atrium from the lungs passes directly across the defect into the right side of the heart. Right ventricular systole therefore takes longer than left ventricular systole and the pulmonary valve closes after the aortic valve throughout, or regardless of the respiratory cycle. As a result, the pulmonary component of the second heart sound always occurs after the aortic component.

Fixed splitting of the second heart sound, as this is known, is an important sign of increased pulmonary blood flow and may be one of the few signs of an atrial septal defect.

Reversed splitting of the second heart sound

Reversed splitting of the second heart sound is an unusual sign that is difficult to hear and is most easily understood by consulting Fig. 7.4 and considering the situation with left bundle branch block.

Owing to the delayed conduction through the left ventricle associated with left bundle branch block, left ventricular systole is late so the aortic valve closes late, as shown in Fig. 7.4. By contrast, the pulmonary valve closes normally, which during inspiration is also late due to extra blood being drawn into the right side of the heart, as explained earlier. Thus, during inspiration, the closure of *both* valves is delayed, with the result that the split between them is narrowed paradoxically, as demonstrated in the figure.

Besides left bundle branch block, reversed splitting of the second heart sound may also be heard in conditions in which conduction through the left ventricle takes longer than normal. Examples of this are the increased mass of ventricular muscle that occurs with aortic stenosis, severe hypertension and cardiomyopathy.

Systolic click

A systolic click is a sound occasionally heard between the first and second heart sounds during ventricular systole, and sounds like 'lub...click...dub'. A click *early* in systole is usually due to the late opening of a stiff stenosed bicuspid aortic valve; a click in the *middle* or *late* in systole is usually a sign of the pathological ballooning of an abnormal cusp of the mitral valve prolapsing up into the left atrium as a result of *mitral valve prolapse.*

Murmurs

Murmurs are sounds due to the *audible vibration* produced by the turbulent flow of blood from a narrow into a wide channel, as illustrated in Fig. 7.5.

A thrill is a palpable vibration, typically produced by a loud murmur.

Some clinicians teach that the way to determine whether a murmur is systolic or diastolic is by timing it against the carotid or radial pulse. Most students, however, find this very difficult. A much easier way of determining both the origin and timing of a murmur is to answer the three following simple questions:

- What does it sound like?

- Where is it loudest?

- Where, if anywhere, does it radiate?

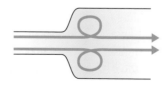

Fig 7.5 Turbulence as blood flows from a narrow to a wide channel

What does it sound like?

● **Systolic murmurs**: All systolic murmurs sound like *Ssssh* or a coarse *Crrrh*. Systolic murmurs also vary in form and length, as illustrated in Fig. 7.6 on page 108, but this does not affect the validity of the method described here for interpreting them, although it can provide information about the severity of the condition and aid interpretation when there are murmurs from more than one valve.

● **Diastolic murmurs**: These are of two types – high-pitch decrescendo murmurs that sound like the clash of a pair of cymbals, *Twwaa* or *Fwirl*, and low-pitch, often barely audible murmurs that sound like a very soft *Urrrh*.

Where is it loudest?

A murmur is usually loudest over the vicinity or downstream from the anatomical position in the chest of the valve responsible for it.

Interpretation of murmurs

The following explanation is in terms of the three questions: what does it sound like, where is it loudest, and where, if anywhere, does it radiate?

Interpreting systolic murmurs

Aortic stenosis

The 2RICS space is downstream from the aortic valve. As a consequence, a harsh systolic *Ssssh* or *Crrrh* murmur that is loudest over the 2RICS, and radiates to the carotid arteries, is classically due to aortic stenosis (Box 7.3) and the turbulence created by blood flowing out through a stenosed aortic valve during ventricular systole.

However, many systolic murmurs in the same or other areas are *innocent flow murmurs*. In the elderly, such a murmur in the 2RICS is often due to *aortic sclerosis*, a condition in which the cusps of the aortic valve move normally and are normal except for fibrotic thickening at their bases. An echocardiogram is the best way of differentiating between innocent and pathological systolic murmurs.

The most common causes of aortic stenosis are calcification of a congenitally bicuspid valve, calcification in old age of a previously normal tricuspid (aortic) valve, and chronic rheumatic valvular disease.

Box 7.3: Clinical features of aortic stenosis

Triad of symptoms
- Chest pain due to angina pectoris
- Breathlessness due to congestion of the lungs caused by left ventricular failure
- Dizziness, syncope (loss of consciousness due to poor cerebral perfusion) or sudden death

Signs
- See Table 7.1 on page 110

Pulmonary stenosis

The 2LICS space is downstream from the pulmonary valve. As a consequence, a systolic murmur loudest over the 2LICS, radiating to the left, is typically due to *pulmonary stenosis* and the turbulence created by blood flowing through a stenosed pulmonary valve during ventricular systole. Pulmonary stenosis is rare but is one of the four features of Fallot's tetralogy (see page 109).

Very occasionally, a soft systolic flow murmur over the 2LICS is one of the few signs of an atrial septal defect.

Mitral regurgitation

Sound from the mitral valve is heard best at the cardiac apex. As a consequence, a systolic murmur loudest at the cardiac apex, radiating to the axilla, is typically due to *mitral regurgitation* and the turbulence created during ventricular systole by blood flowing back into the left atrium through an incompetent leaky mitral valve.

The most common causes of mitral regurgitation are dilatation of the atrioventricular ring due to left ventricular failure, rupture or stretch of a papillary muscle following myocardial infarction, chronic rheumatic valvular disease or infective endocarditis.

VSD

The ventricular septum lies underneath the lower left sternal edge. As a consequence, a systolic murmur that is loudest over the lower left sternal edge is typically due to a VSD and the turbulence created by blood flowing from the high-pressure left ventricle into the low-pressure right ventricle during ventricular systole.

A VSD is most commonly either congenital or due to rupture of the interventricular septum following myocardial infarction.

Interpreting diastolic murmurs

Whereas, as explained above, many systolic murmurs are innocent flow murmurs, all diastolic murmurs are pathological.

Aortic regurgitation

The direction of the flow of blood in aortic regurgitation is back into the heart and down along the left sternal edge during diastole. As a consequence, a high-pitch diastolic murmur that sounds like the clash of a pair of cymbals, *Twwaa* or *Fwirl*, and is loudest over the left sternal edge, is usually due to aortic regurgitation.

The most common causes of aortic regurgitation are chronic rheumatic valvular disease, a collagenosis, infective endocarditis, dilatation of the aortic ring due to severe hypertension or, rarely, prolapse of the valve into a VSD.

Pulmonary regurgitation

The direction of the flow of blood in pulmonary regurgitation is back into the heart and down along the left sternal edge during diastole. As a consequence, a high-pitch diastolic murmur that is similar to the murmur of aortic regurgitation and sounds like the clash of a pair of cymbals, *Twwaa* or *Fwirl*, and is loudest over the left sternal edge, is *very occasionally* due to pulmonary regurgitation, which is much less common than aortic regurgitation. When it occurs, pulmonary regurgitation is typically caused by dilatation of the valvular ring due to pulmonary hypertension.

> ### Note!
>
> *The murmur of aortic regurgitation.* The diastolic murmur of aortic regurgitation is usually accompanied by a systolic murmur that may be due to accompanying aortic stenosis or may be an innocent flow murmur due to the increased stoke-volume associated with aortic regurgitation.
>
> The explanation of the increased stroke volume associated with aortic regurgitation is that blood flowing back normally from the lungs to the heart is joined in the left ventricle by the blood that has regurgitated back through the incompetent valve.
>
> Thus, in a patient at rest, if 70 ml of blood flows back into the left ventricle from the lungs, to be joined by 40 ml of regurgitant blood, the heart will pump out 70 + 40 = 110 ml, which is considerably greater that the normal stroke volume of about 70 ml and enough to create a systolic flow murmur.

Mitral stenosis

The mitral valve is heard best at the cardiac apex. As a consequence, a low-pitch rumbling diastolic *Urrrh* murmur loudest at the apex is usually due to blood flowing in diastole from the left atrium into the left ventricle through a stenosed mitral valve. The most common cause of mitral stenosis is chronic rheumatic valvular disease or rarely an atrial myxoma.

Note!

Mitral stenosis. Because the valve is stiff, it takes longer to open than normal, and when it does so, it is with a high-pitch snap known as an *opening snap*. As demonstrated in Fig. 7.6, this occurs early in diastole, before the murmur, and is immediately after the aortic and pulmonary valves have closed and created the second heart sound. On auscultation, the heart sounds + opening snap + murmur of mitral stenosis sound like *lub, dub, der, urrrh*.

The murmur of mitral stenosis is most easily heard by applying the bell of the stethoscope *very lightly* against the chest wall. Very occasionally, however, a similar sounding rumble without an opening snap may be heard at the apex in *aortic regurgitation*. This is the *Austin Flint murmur* and is due to fluttering of the anterior cusp of the mitral valve as blood regurgitates past it on its way back into the heart during diastole.

Note!

A summary of the different types of murmur is illustrated in Fig. 7.6.

Pericardial rub

A pericardial rub is due to the two surfaces of an inflamed pericardium rubbing together in both systole and diastole to produce what may be mistaken for a systolic murmur followed by a diastolic murmur in the vicinity of the left sternal edge. However, the two components of a pericardial rub are usually much coarser and 'closer' to the ears than a murmur and typically sound like the grating of sandpaper.

A pericardial rub is most commonly caused by viral infection, myocardial infarction, or Dressler's syndrome – an uncommon autoimmune reaction due to cardiac antigens released into the

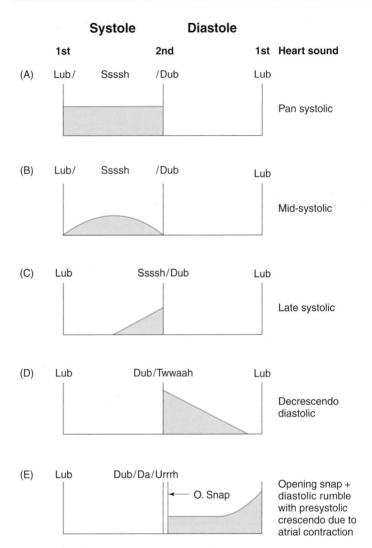

Fig 7.6 Diagrammatic representation of murmurs. (A) Pansystolic. (B) Mid-systolic. (C) Late systolic. (D) Decrescendo diastolic. (E) Opening snap and diastolic rumble with presystolic crescendo due to atrial contraction

blood, most commonly after myocardial infarction, trauma to the heart or viral pericarditis.

Box 7.4 lists signs of important congenital cardiac conditions causing a murmur.

Box 7.4: Signs of rare but important congenital cardiac conditions causing murmurs

Tetralogy of Fallot
- *Reminder of the pathology*: large ventricular septal defect, pulmonary stenosis, aorta overriding both the left and right ventricles, right ventricular hypertrophy
- *Signs*: dyspnoea, cyanosis, clubbing of the fingers, polycythaemia, sternal heave but normal-size heart, systolic murmur due to pulmonary stenosis ± thrill; characteristic squatting position at rest

Patent ductus arteriosus
- *Reminder of the pathology*: failure of the ductus arteriosus (the connection between the pulmonary artery and the aorta in the fetus) to close after birth
- *Signs*: bounding pulse, low diastolic blood pressure, hyperdynamic laterally displaced apex, continuous 'machinery' murmur with both systolic and diastolic components over the second left intercostal space ± thrill

Coarctation of the aorta
- *Reminder of the pathology*: congenital narrowing of the aorta, most commonly below the origin of the left subclavian artery
- *Signs*: low blood pressure and relative ischaemia of the lower half of the body, causing cool legs and claudication, usually with hypertension in the upper half of the body; absent or reduced femoral pulse with delay when palpated simultaneously with the radial pulse; systolic bruit (due to the narrowing) heard over the front and back of the chest; visible collateral vessels on the back accompanied by a soft continuous humming flow-sound throughout both systole and diastole

Table 7.1 Summary of cardiac signs

	Aortic stenosis	Mitral regurgitation	Aortic regurgitation	Mitral stenosis	Congestive cardiac failure	Atrial septal defect
Pulse	Slow rising, small volume	Normal or jerky	Waterhammer ± pulsus bisferiens	Small volume	Normal, or small volume with very severe disease	Usually normal
Jugular venous pulse	Normal ± large 'a' wave	Normal unless raised due to pulmonary hypertension and right heart failure	Normal ± carotid pulsation known as Corrigan's sign	Normal	Raised	Usually normal
Apex (observation and palpation)	Sustained forceful in normal position or a little displaced ± double apex	Hyperdynamic, or possibly sustained and displaced laterally	Hyperdynamic ± displaced downwards and laterally with severe disease	Normal position or inside mid-clavicular line, often with a tapping quality	Sustained and displaced laterally	Usually normal
Sternum (observation and palpation)	Nil of note	Parasternal heave with or without pulmonary hypertension	Nil of note	Parasternal heave if pulmonary hypertension present	Parasternal heave	Right ventricular sternal heave often present

Heart sounds	Absent or soft single A_2 sound in the second right intercostal space	Often a third heart sound	Second heart sound often inaudible because of murmur ± third heart sound	Loud or alternatively soft first heart sound at the apex plus opening snap due to mitral valve opening late after the second heart sound	Fourth heart sound ± third heart sound	Wide fixed splitting of the second heart sound
Thrills and murmurs	Systolic thrill in second right intercostal space with severe disease Coarse systolic murmur in second right intercostal space radiating to the carotids	Apical thrill with severe disease Systolic murmur radiating to the axilla	Thrill occasionally along left sternal edge with severe disease Decrescendo diastolic murmur at left sternal edge	Apical diastolic thrill with severe disease and patient lying over to the left Apical diastolic rumble plus presystolic accentuation due to atrial contraction in patients in sinus rhythm	Murmur possible, depending on the cause of the congestive cardiac failure and its consequences, such as dilatation of the atrio-ventricular ring producing a murmur of mitral regurgitation	Usually no murmur from the atrial septal defect itself ± systolic flow murmur in pulmonary artery over second left intercostal space ± mid-diastolic rumble along left sternal edge due to increased blood flow through the tricuspid valve

8

PERIPHERAL VASCULAR SYSTEM

EXAMINATION

Hands and arms

Inspection

● Ask the patient to extend both hands and arms in the supine position.

● Compare both hands and arms simultaneously for rashes, changes in the texture of the skin, scars, venous pattern, colour (whiteness suggests ischaemia; blueness may be due to either ischaemia or cyanosis), swelling, symmetry, oedema and hair distribution (loss of hair may be due to ischaemia or peripheral neuropathy).

Palpation

Capillary refilling time

● Depress the skin on the distal pad of a finger and observe the time taken for the colour to return; this is normally 2–3 seconds.

Temperature

● The most sensitive way of assessing temperature is with the backs of your fingers.

● Feel the palms and then the flexor surfaces of both the patient's arms simultaneously up to his biceps muscles with the backs of your fingers, noting any coolness suggestive of impaired circulation or unusual warmth suggestive of inflammation or venous congestion.

Pulses

● Use two or three fingers of each hand to simultaneously palpate and compare the strength of the two radial pulses.

● Then palpate the brachial pulse in one arm by slightly flexing the patient's arm and palpating in the fold of the elbow slightly to the medial side of the biceps tendon with either your thumb or index and middle fingers.

Allen test

● This test is used to assess the arterial blood supply to the hand.

● Ask the patient to place his hand in the supine position.

● Now place your thumbs lightly over the radial and ulnar pulses just above the wrist.

- Ask the patient to make a tight fist in order to squeeze blood from it.

- Tightly compress both arteries with your thumbs.

- Ask the patient to open his hand. The palm should be pale due to lack of blood.

- Release the pressure over the ulnar artery. If the artery is patent, the palm should flush and become pink within 3–5 seconds.

- Repeat the procedure for the radial artery.

Lymph nodes

- Palpate the *epitrochlear nodes* by supporting the patient's arm with one of your hands and palpating with your other hand in the groove between the biceps and triceps muscles on the medial side of the arm about 3 or 4 cm above the medial epicondyle.

- Note the size, consistency and any tenderness of the nodes, although they are normally palpable only in patients with marked infection of the distal arm.

Legs

Inspection

- Compare one leg with the other from the groins to the toes for symmetry, rashes, changes in the texture of the skin, scars, venous pattern, colour (duskiness of the feet and lower legs suggests ischaemia), ulcers, oedema and hair distribution (loss of hair may occur with ischaemia or peripheral neuropathy).

Note!

Background information about ulcers on the legs is on page 118.

Varicose veins

● Ask the patient to stand, and look for any abnormal venous swelling suggestive of varicose veins (mainly on the backs of the legs).

Palpation

This is performed with the patient lying in the supine position.

Capillary refilling time

● Assess capillary refilling time on the dorsum of the big toe of both feet, using the method described on page 113 for the arms.

Temperature

● Assess the temperature of the feet, shins and thighs of both legs simultaneously, using the method described on page 113 for the arms.

Pulses

● **Femoral pulse:** use the tips of two or three fingers of your right hand to palpate slightly to the medial side of the centre of the groin beneath the inguinal ligament.

● **Popliteal pulse:** ask the patient to flex his hip and knee but keep his foot on the table. Then place your thumbs on the top of the front of the tibia and identify the pulse by pressing firmly with the fingers of both hands behind the partially flexed knee. Identifying this pulse may be difficult but may be made easier by asking the patient to roll over into the prone position with his knee flexed to 90° and his foot resting on your shoulder.

● **Posterior tibial pulse:** this is most easily palpated by curling the index, middle and ring fingers of your right hand around the back of the *medial malleolus.*

● **Dorsalis pedis pulse:** this pulse is usually located in the *middle* of the dorsum of the foot, *lateral* to the long extensor tendon to the big toe.

> ### Note!
>
> All four foot pulses are usually present. However, many healthy people have only one palpable pulse in each foot, or one in one foot and two in the other.

Lymph nodes

● Use the tips of two or three fingers of your right hand to palpate the *inguinal lymph nodes* as they lie along the inguinal ligament, and the *femoral lymph nodes* as they lie in the femoral canal, medial to the femoral vein, the position of which is described on page 281.

> ### Note!
>
> Background information about abnormalities of the lymph nodes in the legs is on page 119.

Oedema

● Press with the tips of the fingers of your right hand for at least 5 seconds over the dorsum of the feet, behind the medial malleoli and over the shins, checking for any visible or palpable indentation.

> ### Note!
>
> Background information about the causes of oedema of the legs is on page 119.

Calves

● Gently squeeze the calves and dorsiflex the foot (Homan's sign), noting any tenderness. Remember that a positive test may be due to either a deep venous thrombosis or a torn calf muscle, and that the test is therefore non-specific and of little value in diagnosing deep venous thrombosis.

Trendelenburg test

● This is a test of the competence of the venous valves in the leg, and is done if venous insufficiency is suspected.

● Ask the patient to lie supine, and then assist him to elevate one leg to 90° for 30 seconds to drain the blood from the veins.

● Occlude the long saphenous vein by *firmly* gripping the *medial side* of the thigh in the angle between your thumb and index finger.

● Ask the patient to stand while maintaining a firm grip over the vein.

● If the superficial veins beneath your hand fill in less than 30 seconds, the perforator veins between the deep and superficial veins are incompetent.

● Release your hand. Further rapid filling of the superficial veins indicates backward filling due to defective valves in the long saphenous vein.

Note!

This test may be difficult to perform and is not very reliable.

Arterial insufficiency

● Ask the patient to lie supine in such a position that his legs can dangle over the end of the table.

● Raise both legs to 60° for 60 seconds. An increase of any pallor of the legs indicates arterial insufficiency.

● Ask the patient to sit up and dangle his legs over the end of the table.

- Return of pinkness taking longer than 10 seconds or filling of the veins in the feet taking longer than 15 seconds indicates arterial insufficiency.

- Dusky redness (rubor) also suggests arterial insufficiency.

The clinical features of ischaemia of the leg are listed in Box 8.1.

> **Box 8.1: Clinical features of ischaemia of the leg**
>
> - Pain in the calf on walking (claudication)
> - Dusky appearance (rubor)
> - Loss of hair on the limb
> - Impaired capillary refilling time
> - Coolness or coldness on palpation
> - Absent foot pulses
> - Peripheral ulcers or gangrene, starting on the toes

Sacrum

- This test is usually done only on patients who are confined to bed or a chair.

- Ask the patient to roll over onto his left side so you can inspect his sacral area for bed sores and test for oedema.

BACKGROUND INFORMATION

Leg ulcers, lymph nodes and oedema of the legs

Ulcers

Ulcers of the lower leg: The most common site of ulcers on the legs is on the *medial side above the medial malleolus.* Conditions predisposing to ulcers at this site include varicose veins, diabetes mellitus, trauma, atherosclerosis and vasculitis.

Neuropathic ulcers of the type seen in diabetes mellitus, occur as a result of friction/pressure under the metatarsal heads and under the toes of a foot that is usually warm and well perfused with palpable pulses and dry skin.

Ischaemic ulcers on the foot occur as a result of atherosclerosis that is usually secondary to diabetes mellitus and/or smoking, and typically occur in the periphery on the ends of the toes and may lead to gangrene in a foot that is cold and pulseless with dry atrophic skin. Similar looking ulcers may occur due to lack of sensation in patients with neuropathy who wear tight shoes.

Ulcers on the heel occur with both neuropathy and ischaemia or a mixture of both.

Inguinal lymph nodes

Small shotty glands may be felt in healthy people. Swollen tender glands suggest infection. Hard, irregular, enlarged glands that are deeply attached suggest metastases from a pelvic carcinoma. Rubbery enlargement of the glands suggests lymphoma.

Oedema

Oedema of the leg may be due to local conditions such as inflammation caused by infection; increased hydrostatic pressure at the venous end of capillaries due typically to varicose veins or right heart failure; and low osmotic pressure at the venous end of the capillaries due to the low-albumin states listed on page 148.

9

RESPIRATORY SYSTEM

Equipment needed

- Stethoscope

Position of the patient

- The patient should be in warm quiet surroundings, either lying or sitting upright during examination of the front of the chest and sitting upright during examination of the back of the chest

Order of the examination

- Inspection
- Palpation
- Percussion
- Auscultation

When examining the chest (or abdomen), always compare one side with the other rather than comparing different areas on the same side.

EXAMINATION

Inspection – initially from the front

General appearance (relevant to the respiratory system)

- Assess the patient for signs of smoker's face (page 34), breathlessness, cyanosis or use of accessory muscles, such as the sternomastoid muscle, the arms or the intercostal muscles.

Respiratory rate

- As explained on page 56, because breathing is under voluntary control and will unwittingly change if the patient is aware that his respiratory rate is being counted, it is best to count the rate while holding the patient's arm and appearing to take the radial pulse.

- Count the movements of the chest as the patient breaths in and out for half a minute and multiple by two, or alternatively count for a minute. In adults, the respiratory rate at rest is normally 14–20 breaths per minute.

Respiratory pattern

- Apart from counting the respiratory rate, also note the *pattern* of breathing.

Note!

Background information about abnormalities in the pattern of breathing is on page 128.

Inspection of the hands (relevant to the respiratory system)

- Look for cyanosis, clubbing and nicotine staining of the fingers. Cyanosis is discussed on page 40, and the causes of finger clubbing are listed on page 47.

Trachea

Inspection

● Inspect the trachea to check whether it appears to be central or deviated to one side or the other.

Palpation

● If you have not already done so as part of the examination of the head and neck, determine whether the trachea is central or deviated to one side or the other by one of the following methods:
  ○ Run a single finger down the centre of the trachea and determine whether it runs through the centre of the suprasternal notch or to the side.
  ○ Run each of your index fingers, or the index and middle fingers of your right hand, down either side of the trachea and determine whether it is central or deviated to the side by referring to the inner ends of the clavicles.

Note!

Background information about deviation of the trachea is on page 129.

Lymph nodes

● If you have not already done so as part of the examination of the head and neck, palpate the supraclavicular lymph nodes on either side of the neck above the clavicle and immediately lateral to the sternomastoid muscle, as carcinoma of the bronchus has a tendency to metastasize to these nodes.

The five sites to which carcinoma of the bronchus commonly metastasize are listed in Box 9.1.

Box 9.1: Five main sites to which carcinoma of the bronchus may metastasize

- Liver
- Bone
- Brain
- Supraclavicular lymph nodes
- Adrenal glands (approximately 4 per cent of cases)

Examination of the thorax

Order of the examination
- First carry out a complete examination of the front of the chest, that is, inspection, palpation, percussion, auscultation.
- Then repeat the complete examination on the back of the chest.

Inspection

Shape of the chest

- Look to see whether both sides of the chest are of equal size, or whether one side is sunken due, for instance, to collapse of the underlying lung.

- Also note whether the ribs have moved closer together on one side as a result of collapse of the underlying lung.

Deformities of the thorax

Look for deformities such as:

- **funnel chest (pectus excavatum)**, in which the sternum is congenitally abnormally sunken;

- **pigeon chest (pectus carinatum)**, in which the sternum is congenitally abnormally prominent and the chest is narrow;

Note: Both the above deformities may occur with Marfan's syndrome.

- **barrel chest**, a common sign of emphysema, in which there is an increase in the anteroposterior diameter of the chest that occurs as a result of the increased volume of the lungs associated with the condition. Barrel chest is most easily assessed by inspecting the patient from the side.

Movements of the thorax

Check the movements of the chest for the following:

- **Equality of the movements on both sides**: usually movements on both sides of the chest are equal. However, owing to the fact that less air enters a side with the following pathologies, movements are less over the side of an effusion, collapse, consolidation or pneumothorax.

- **Flail chest**: If the patient has suffered trauma to the chest, check for paradoxical movement caused by the ribs on *both* sides of the chest being fractured, with the result that the sternum and centre of the chest are *drawn in* rather than moving out as the patient inspires. Flail chest typically results from a road traffic accident in which the patient's chest hit the steering wheel of a car.

Palpation

Tenderness

- Compare one side of the chest with the other at three or four levels by gently pressing with the pads of the fingers of your right hand, first on one side and then the other. Alternatively, use both hands to press on both sides simultaneously.

Note!

Tenderness over the chest may be due to trauma, pulled muscles and minor cracks in the ribs associated with osteoporosis, particularly in middle-aged and elderly women. Tenderness may also occasionally be associated with underlying pleurisy or metastases in the ribs.

Expansion of the thorax

● Check expansion of the lower half of the chest by placing both your hands symmetrically over either side of the lower chest with your thumbs and fingers spread widely apart and pointing laterally.

● Now ask the patient to inspire deeply while you watch the movement of your hands. Movement is normally equal on both sides.

● Repeat at the top of the chest.

● Because less air enters a side with the following pathologies, expansion is decreased over the side of an effusion, collapse, consolidation or pneumothorax.

Tactile fremitus

● Tactile fremitus is a vibration felt on the surface of the chest as the patient speaks.

● Compare one side of the chest with the other at three or four levels by placing the fingers of your right hand flat on the chest to feel for vibrations, first on one side and then on the other, as the patient says 'ninety-nine'.

● Alternatively, instead of using your fingers alone, you may use the fingers and palm combined or the medial edge of your hand; instead of placing one hand at a time on the chest, you may alternatively use both hands to test both sides simultaneously.

> **Note!**
>
> Background information about abnormalities affecting tactile fremitus is on page 137 and in Table 9.1 on page 139.

Percussion of the thorax

● Percussion is performed by placing and spreading the fingers of your non-dominant hand on the patient's chest and tapping the terminal digit or nail of its middle finger with the tip of the terminal digit of the middle finger of your dominant hand, as if striking with a hammer (Fig. 9.1). Alternatively, you may percuss with both the index and middle fingers of your dominant hand. The best results of percussion are obtained by semiflexing the joints of the percussing finger or fingers so that the distal phalange is vertical at the moment of impact, as illustrated in Fig. 9.1, and by making the movements of your hand mainly at the wrist.

● Start percussing above the clavicles, and compare one side with the other at about five levels, moving downwards in the mid-clavicular line. In addition, at the base of the chest, percuss at two levels in the mid-axillary line, so that on each side of the chest you end up having percussed roughly in the shape of a 'J' or backward 'J'.

● The quality of the sound that results varies with the nature of the underlying contents of the chest and is discussed on page 137 and in Table 9.1 (page 139).

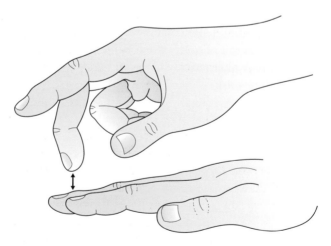

Fig 9.1 Percussing with the middle finger

● **Diaphragmatic movement**: When examining the back of the chest, assess diaphragmatic movement by asking the patient to *exhale* and hold his breath for a few seconds while you percuss over the lower half of one side of his chest to determine the lowest level of resonance. Mark the level with a ballpoint pen. Then repeat the procedure after the patient has *inhaled* and is holding his breath for another few seconds. The difference between the two levels is the diaphragmatic movement, which is normally between 5–6 cm. If necessary, repeat on the other side.

Auscultation

Breath sounds

● Start above the clavicles and listen with the diaphragm of the stethoscope to both inspiration and expiration, first on one side of the chest and then on the other, at about five levels, moving downwards in the mid-clavicular line. In addition, at the bases of the lungs listen at two levels in the mid-axillary line, so that on each side of the chest you end up having auscultated roughly in the shape of a 'J' or backward 'J'.

● Note the quality of the breath sounds, and whether they are normal, reduced or bronchial. In addition, listen for added sounds, such as crackles and wheezes, all of which are discussed on page 133 and in Table 9.1, on page 139.

Vocal fremitus

● Vocal fremitus is similar to tactile fremitus but is heard with the diaphragm of the stethoscope rather than being felt with the hand. Vocal fremitus is demonstrated by asking the patient to repeatedly say 'ninety-nine' and comparing the quality of the sound heard on one side of the chest with the quality on the other side at about four or five levels, moving downwards in the mid-clavicular line. In addition, at the base of the lung listen at one or two levels in the mid-axillary line so that on each side of the chest you end up having listened roughly in the shape of a 'J' or backward 'J'.

Note!

Background information about abnormalities of vocal fremitus is on page 137 and in Table 9.1 (page 139).

BACKGROUND INFORMATION

Respiratory pattern

An uncomfortable awareness of breathing is known as *dyspnoea* and is seen in many conditions such as left heart failure and respiratory diseases such as chronic obstructive pulmonary disease (COPD; Box 9.2), bronchial asthma, pleural effusion, pneumothorax and pneumonia.

Box 9.2: Clinical features of chronic obstructive pulmonary disease

Symptoms
- None (early disease), *or*:
- Sputum production
- Breathlessness on exertion
- Swelling of the ankles due to right heart failure, secondary to pulmonary hypertension caused by chronic anoxia (predominantly bronchitic disease)
- Drowsiness/confusion secondary to carbon dioxide retention (predominantly bronchitic disease)
- Association with smoking

Signs
- Smoker's face (page 34)
- Respiratory distress
- Increased respiratory rate and breathlessness with prolonged expiration
- Wheeze

- Central cyanosis (predominantly bronchitic disease)
- Use of accessory muscles of respiration
- Barrel chest (predominantly emphysematous disease)
- Reduced breath sounds due to narrowed airways
- Peripheral oedema (see previous page for mechanism)
- Drowsiness/confusion (see previous page for mechanism)

In asthma and COPD, expiration takes longer than normal, as the airways are pathologically narrow and the increase in intrathoracic pressure that occurs during *expiration* compresses them even further, with the result that it takes longer to breathe out than normal.

In metabolic acidosis, the breathing is regular but has a *deep sighing* quality known as *Kussmaul breathing* that occurs as a result of carbon dioxide being blown off to compensate for the loss of bicarbonate associated with the acidosis, as per the Henderson/Hasselbalch equation.

Although the pattern of breathing is usually regular, it is occasionally irregular, consisting of a period of deep sighing breaths followed by a period of apnoea. This is known as *Cheyne-Stokes respiration* and is due to *altered sensitivity of the respiratory centre* caused by ischaemia resulting from a stroke or heart failure. What happens is that, during the periods of deep sighing, the patient blows off abnormal amounts of carbon dioxide, resulting in a low arterial partial pressure of carbon dioxide and low carbon dioxide drive to the respiratory centre. As a consequence, breathing becomes slow and shallow and then stops for a few seconds until the arterial partial pressure of carbon dioxide has built up enough again to drive the respiratory centre, and the cycle repeats itself.

Deviation of the trachea

Deviation of the trachea is a useful sign for differentiating between four of the main pathologies of the lung, namely collapse, effusion, consolidation and pneumothorax.

Collapse of a lung or part of a lung and pleural effusion

Collapse occurs as the result of blockage of a bronchus. As a consequence, air no longer enters the lung, and the lung shrinks and collapses as the air that is already in it is absorbed into the bloodstream. The effect on the trachea of the lung becoming smaller is to *pull the trachea towards the side of the collapse.*

By contrast, *pleural effusion*, which is defined as fluid between the parietal and visceral layers of the pleura, increases the contents of the thorax. When this is unilateral, its effect on the trachea is *to push the trachea away from the side of the effusion*, that is towards the *opposite* side of the chest.

Consolidation

Consolidation is usually caused by pneumonia. In this situation, the alveoli are full of inflammatory cells and exudate, but the size of the lung is unaffected so the trachea remains in its normal midline position.

Pneumothorax

Pneumothorax is air between the two layers of the pleura and may have one of two effects on the trachea. With a *spontaneous pneumothorax*, the lung collapses until the hole closes and the situation stabilizes with the lung partially or completely collapsed and air in the pleural space and the trachea and mediastinum in their central position. By contrast, as explained on page 132, with a *tension pneumothorax* the pressure within the pneumothorax increases rapidly and pushes the trachea to the *opposite* side of the chest.

Causes of collapse of a lung, pleural effusion and pneumothorax

Collapse

The most common cause of collapse of a lung or part of a lung is carcinoma blocking a bronchus, although occasionally a mucous plug or an inhaled foreign body such as a peanut may also cause it.

Pleural effusion

Two types of pleural effusion are recognized, namely transudate and exudate.

Transudate is due to fluid not being drawn back into the circulation from the surface of the pleura. Transudates are caused by raised hydrostatic pressure at the venous end of capillaries (such as occurs with left heart failure) or low osmotic pressure at the venous end of the capillaries due to hypoalbuminaemia resulting from any of the conditions listed on page 148. The protein content of an transudate is typically less than 30 g/L.

Exudate is due to protein-rich fluid oozing into the pleural space as a result of the pleura being inflamed by conditions such as pneumonia, carcinoma of the bronchus (Boxes 9.3 and 9.4) or mesothelioma. The protein content of an exudate is typically over 30 g/L, and the lactate dehydrogenase level is abnormally high by comparison with the level in the serum.

Box 9.3: Symptoms of carcinoma of the bronchus

- None (chance finding on chest X-ray), *or:*
- Unwellness due to tumour bulk, metastases or inappropriate antidiuretic hormone secretion
- Cough (change of an established cough or a new cough)
- Coughing blood (haemoptysis)
- Breathlessness due to tumour bulk, collapse of the lung, pleural effusion or rarely anaemia
- Weight loss due to poor appetite and toxic effects of tumour
- Pain due to hepatic or bony metastases or pleural invasion
- Facial swelling due to superior vena cava syndrome
- Association with smoking

> **Box 9.4: Signs of carcinoma of the bronchus**
>
> - None, *or*:
> - Cachexia (wasting)
> - Clubbing of the fingers (page 46)
> - Collapse or partial collapse of a lung or pleural effusion
> - Enlarged liver due to metastases
> - Tenderness over bony and hepatic metastases
> - Enlarged supraclavicular lymph nodes
> - Other signs: Horner's syndrome (page 181); facial swelling due to superior vena cava syndrome; atrial fibrillation, pleural or pericardial rub due to invasion of the serous membranes; rarely, hot tender ankles and wrists due to periostitis caused by hypertrophic pulmonary osteoarthropathy

Spontaneous pneumothorax

In this condition, air enters the lung through a hole in the visceral pleura caused by the rupture of a bleb or bulla on or against the surface of the pleura.

Traumatic pneumothorax

Occasionally, a wound to the thorax, such as a knife wound, may allow air into the pleural space through the chest wall. Alternatively, the sharp end of a fractured rib may pierce the visceral pleura and allow air in.

If considerable bleeding occurs, a *haemopneumothorax* may ensue, with blood collecting like an effusion in the dependent part of the chest beneath the pneumothorax.

Tension pneumothorax

As stated on page 130, with most pneumothoraces the trachea remains in its central position. However, the hole that has produced the pneumothorax occasionally acts as a one-way valve that allows air to enter the pleural space each time the patient inspires, but closes as the lung is compressed during expiration. As a result, air cannot escape and the pressure inside the pleural space rapidly increases, leading to a rapid increase in the size of the pneumothorax and life-threatening compression of the contents of the thorax.

This condition is known as a *tension pneumothorax* and is a medical emergency that, as long as the diagnosis has been established with certainty, may be relieved by inserting an intravenous cannula through the chest wall to let the air out.

Breath sounds and added sounds

Breath sounds

Breath sounds are generated by vibrations that occur as air rushes turbulently along large airways. The resulting sound contains a wide spectrum of wavelengths ranging from high to low frequencies. Normal lung filters out the high-frequency sounds, leaving only the low-frequency sounds to reach the surface of the lung and the stethoscope.

Normal breath sounds

As implied in the previous paragraph, normal breath sounds are much quieter than breath sounds heard over a large airway such as the trachea. Another characteristic of the breath sounds is that inspiration normally lasts longer than expiration. In addition, the breath sounds vary slightly from area to area, hence terms such as *vesicular* and *broncho-vesicular*. Such differences are normally, however, of no clinical significance.

Bronchial breathing

Bronchial breathing is loud and similar to the sounds heard over a large airway such as the trachea. Bronchial breathing occurs over areas of consolidation, and is due to the fact that *consolidated lung does not filter out the high-pitch sounds generated in the large airways*, but instead conducts them to the surface along with the low-pitch sounds that are conducted normally.

The consolidation responsible for bronchial breathing is most commonly caused by pneumonia, although it may also occasionally be caused by dense fibrosis.

For an illustration of the difference between normal breath sounds and simulated bronchial breathing, listen with the diaphragm of your stethoscope, first over your own trachea and then over your own lung fields.

Whispering pectoriloquy and bronchophony

Whispering pectoriloquy is a particularly loud response to a very soft whisper. To elicit whispering pectoriloquy, ask the patient to whisper 'ninety-nine' *very softly*. Whispering pectoriloquy is present if you hear the word 'ninety-nine.'

Bronchophony is increased intensity and clarity of the voice when the patient speaks at normal volume. Like bronchial breathing, whispering pectoriloquy and bronchophony are heard over areas of consolidation but not over normal lung, and are due to the conduction of both low- and high-frequency sounds to the stethoscope.

Aegophony

Aegophony is a bleating or high-pitch nasal quality to the voice that results in 'ay' sounding like 'ee.' Aegophony is heard over lung that is compressed by an effusion.

Added sounds

Four types of additional sound are recognized. These are *crackles, wheezes, pleural rub* and *stridor*. Terms such as ronchi, rales and crepitations are confusing and are no longer often used.

Crackles

Crackles are *numerous, almost instantaneous, popping sounds* that occur during *inspiration* and sound somewhat like dozens or hundreds of raindrops plopping onto water or onto the canvas of a tent. Physiologically, crackles are due to small pathologically closed airways popping open as air rushes into them; they are heard in consolidation due to pneumonia, congestion due to left ventricular failure, pulmonary fibrosis (e.g. cryptogenic fibrosing alveolitis), bronchiectasis and occasionally asthma and COPD.

Wheeze

Wheezes are *abnormal continuous sounds that last for a few seconds during expiration*, although in very severe asthma they may also occasionally occur during inspiration. Wheezes are sometimes almost musical, as if made by a reed or horn instrument. Wheezes are due to the walls of pathologically narrowed airways opening and closing very rapidly and, as a consequence, vibrating as air rushes along them. Wheezes occur in asthma, COPD, and sometimes in left ventricular failure as a result of oedema pathologically narrowing the airways.

The clinical features of bronchial asthma are listed in Box 9.5.

Box 9.5: Clinical features of bronchial asthma

Four cardinal symptoms
- Cough
- Wheeze
- Breathlessness
- Tightness in the chest

Signs
- Respiratory distress
- Increased respiratory rate and breathlessness with prolonged, difficult expiration
- Wheeze
- Central cyanosis
- Use of accessory muscles of ventilation
- Sinus tachycardia
- Pulsus paradoxus (page 65)

Pleural rub

Pleural rub is a *crumpling sound* like the crumpling of tissue paper. A pleural rub may be heard when the pleura are inflamed and its two inflamed surfaces rub together as the patient breathes. A pleural rub may occur in many conditions including viral infection, bacterial infection causing pneumonia, invasion by carcinoma of the bronchus, pulmonary embolism or Dressler's syndrome (page 107).

The clinical features of pulmonary embolus are listed in Box 9.6.

Box: 9.6 Clinical features of pulmonary embolus

Peripheral embolus
- Breathlessness
- Haemoptysis due to infarction of lung
- Pleuritic chest pain and a pleural rub due to involvement of the pleura
- Pyrexia (often spikes of temperature)

Central embolus (embolus obstructing a large pulmonary artery)
- Sudden breathlessness and circulatory collapse with a rapid small-volume pulse and low blood pressure
- Central cyanosis
- Jugular venous pressure markedly raised due to central obstruction of the circulation
- Sternal heave due to acute right heart strain
- Gallop third and fourth heart sounds and wide fixed splitting of the second heart sound

---

Stridor

Stridor is a *continuous, high-pitch sound that occurs during inspiration and is like a high-pitch 'inspiratory wheeze'.* Stridor is fairly uncommon in adults and is due to vibrations set up by partial blockage of a large airway, such as the trachea or a main bronchus, most commonly by a proximal carcinoma of the bronchus.

Summary of the various abnormal signs in the chest (see also Table 9.1)

Percussion

Collapse, consolidation and effusion

Collapse of a lung results in the area involved becoming denser or more solid than normal. Effusion and consolidation are also dense. As a result, percussion over areas of collapse, consolidation and effusion tend to be similar, that is, *dull*, although the fluid associated with an effusion is so dense that percussion over an area of effusion is often said to be 'stony dull'.

Pneumothorax and emphysema

Because a pneumothorax contains only air, and emphysema consists of abnormally large air spaces, percussion over these abnormalities is *abnormally resonant.*

Breath sounds, tactile and vocal fremitus

Effusion and pneumothorax

Both an effusion and a pneumothorax act like a blanket or insulating layer around the lung. As a consequence of this and the collapse of the lung associated with them, less sound is conducted to the surface, and the breath sounds, tactile fremitus and vocal fremitus are *reduced.*

Collapse

With collapse of a lung or part of a lung, less air enters the affected side; as a consequence, the intensity of the breath sounds, tactile fremitus and vocal fremitus are *reduced.*

Consolidation

With consolidation, the whole spectrum of sound generated in the trachea is conducted to the surface of the lung, and as a result the breath sounds, tactile fremitus and vocal fremitus are *increased*, with the breath sounds being called *bronchial breathing.*

COPD

In COPD, the airways are pathologically narrow, and the resistance to the flow of air along them is increased. As a result, the rate at which air flows along them is reduced and the breath sounds are *reduced* (quiet). In addition, because of the compression of the airways that occurs during expiration, expiration is prolonged and takes longer than inspiration.

By noting the part of the chest in which the signs described in this section and in Table 9.1 are observed, and by using the information contained in Fig. 9.2, it is an easy matter to work out the lobe or lobes, or part of the lung, in which pathology such as consolidation, collapse, pneumothorax and pleural effusion has occurred.

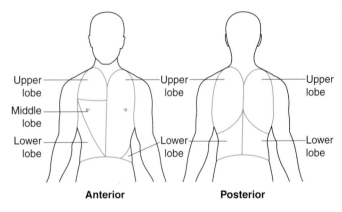

Fig 9.2 Surface boundaries of the lobes of the lungs

Table 9.1 Summary of respiratory signs

	Collapse	Effusion	Consolidation	Pneumothorax	COPD, predominantly chronic bronchitis	COPD, predominantly emphysema
Common cause	Carcinoma	Carcinoma or heart failure	Pneumonia	Torn pleural ruptured bleb or bulla	Smoking	Smoking
Trachea	Towards	Away	Central	Usually central Away with a tension pneumothorax	Central	Central
Percussion	Dull	Dull	Dull	Hyperresonant	Normal	Hyperresonant
Tactile Fremitus	Decreased	Decreased	Increased	Decreased	Normal or decreased	Decreased
Breath Sounds	Decreased	Decreased	Increased, i.e. bronchial	Decreased	Decreased + prolonged expiration	Decreased + prolonged expiration
Vocal Fremitus	Decreased	Decreased	Increased	Decreased	Normal or decreased	Decreased

COPD, chronic obsctructive pulmonary disease.

10

ABDOMINAL SYSTEM

Equipment needed

- Stethoscope
- Glove and tube of lubricant

Position of the patient

- The patient should be lying in warm, quiet surroundings with a cover over his legs and inguinal regions, and in the case of a female patient, over the breasts, except when percussing the upper border of the liver
- Observe the patient's face for pain whenever you touch his abdomen.

Order of the examination

- Inspection
- Auscultation
- Percussion
- Palpation

EXAMINATION

Inspection

Face (relevant to the abdominal system)

● Inspect the face to see whether the patient appears to be in pain, and also whether there is jaundice, anaemia (caused, for instance, by loss of blood from the gastrointestinal tract or malabsorption), dehydration (caused, for instance, by vomiting or diarrhoea) or angular cheilitis (page 72).

Hands (relevant to the abdominal system)

● Inspect the hands for anaemia and clubbing (associated with cirrhosis of the liver, ulcerative colitis and Crohn's disease), and for palmar erythema and Dupuytren's contracture (associated with excessive alcohol intake).

Abdomen

● Inspect the abdomen for abnormalities of its contours, for example because of distension caused by any of the five Fs (fat, faeces, flatus, fluid or fetus) or masses, organomegaly or distension of the bladder.

● Note any scars, hernias, abnormally dilated veins (due to portal hypertension resulting from cirrhosis of the liver), striae, spider naevi (both of which are described in the Note in the next paragraph), or lack of movement due to rigidity caused by inflammation of the peritoneum.

> ## Note!
>
> An *abdominal hernia* is an abnormal protrusion of tissue through the abdominal wall. Such a hernia may be inguinal, umbilical or incisional. *Striae* are stretch marks or depressed streaks in the skin, usually due to obesity or pregnancy.

Spider naevi are small dilated blood vessels that consist of a central vessel with slender vessels resembling the legs of a spider radiating out from the centre. Spiders, as they are often known, occur in the distribution of the superior vena cava and blanche on pressure. One or two may be seen occasionally in healthy people, particularly in pregnancy. More are typical of chronic liver disease, the signs of which are listed in Box 10.1.

Box 10.1: Signs of chronic liver disease

General appearance
- Remnants of blood due to vomiting from bleeding varices or peptic ulcer
- Atrophic skin and thin limbs due to poor nutrition
- Jaundice
- Bruising
- Spider naevi due to failure to metabolize oestrogens

Hands
- Flapping tremor if hepatic encephalopathy is present (page 38)
- Palmar erythema (page 50)
- Dupuytren's contracture (page 49)
- Minor clubbing of the fingers (page 46)

Trunk
- Gynaecomastia in the male
- Dilated veins over the abdomen and lower chest due to congestion caused by portal hypertension
- Either an enlarged or a small liver, depending upon the cause and stage of the disease
- Enlarged spleen if portal hypertension is present
- Feminization of hair distribution and testicular atrophy in the male

Auscultation

Use the diaphragm of the stethoscope to auscultate for the following.

Bowel sounds

- These can be difficult to hear. Listen in the centre of the abdomen for tinkling sounds, which are due to peristalsis causing the contents of the bowel to move.

- If bowel sounds are difficult to hear, try listening over each quadrant of the abdomen.

Renal bruits

- Auscultate bilaterally in the upper quadrants of the abdomen about 7–8 cm from the midline and 2–3 cm or so below the lowest rib. If necessary, make allowance for the shape of the rib cage. (Bruits are described on page 82.)

Other bruits

- If you suspect ischaemia of the legs, listen slightly to the left of the umbilicus for a bruit over the aorta. Also listen in the centres of the left and right lower abdominal quadrants for bruits from the iliac arteries, and just medial to and beneath the centre of the inguinal ligaments for bruits over the pulsation of the femoral arteries.

Note!

Background information about abnormalities of the bowel sounds and the implications of renal bruits is on page 154.

Percussion

- The technique for percussing the abdomen is the same as the technique for percussing the chest, and is described on page 125.

- First, percuss all four quadrants, *comparing one side with the other* for any dullness that might indicate a mass, enlarged organ, faeces or fluid (due either to ascites or blood in the peritoneal cavity (*haemoperitoneum*)).

- In addition, as you percuss, note any tenderness that may indicate inflammation of the peritoneum or abnormal distension and hyperresonance suggesting intestinal obstruction, the clinical features of which are listed in Box 10.2. The most common cause of intestinal obstruction is cancer of the bowel, the clinical features of which are listed in Box 10.3.

Box 10.2: Clinical features of intestinal obstruction

Symptoms
- Feeling unwell
- Colicky abdominal pain
- Nausea, vomiting
- Constipation and absence of flatus (wind)
- Abdominal distension

Signs
- Abdominal distension and hyperresonance on percussion
- Increased bowel sounds
- Tenderness if there is inflamed or strangulated bowel
- Rectal examination: often empty, i.e. absence of stool

Box 10.3: Clinical features of cancer of the bowel

Symptoms
- None; result of screening for occult blood in the stool, sigmoidoscopy or colonoscopy, or:
- Loss of appetite and weight loss
- Alteration of bowel habit, with either constipation or increased frequency of stool
- Abdominal pain with left-sided cancer
- Rectal bleeding with sigmoid and rectal cancer
- Asymptomatic iron deficiency anaemia with cancer in the caecum or right side of the colon

Signs
- None, *or*:
- Anaemia (page 33)
- Gauntness and evidence of loss of weight
- Palpable mass
- Hepatomegaly due to hepatic metastases
- Blood and/or a palpable mass on rectal examination
- Signs of intestinal obstruction (see Box 10.2)

Liver

- **Lower border:** Start percussing in the right lower quadrant of the abdomen, as the liver may be unexpectedly large. Work upwards towards the right lower ribs, noting the level at which any dullness occurs

- **Upper border:** Start high up in the chest in the mid-clavicular line, well above the level of the nipple in a man, and work downwards, noting the level at which dullness occurs

- The size of the liver on percussion in the mid-clavicular line is normally between 6 and 12 cm. The causes of a large liver are listed in Box 10.4.

Box 10.4: Causes of a large liver or an apparently large liver

- **Anatomic**, e.g.:
  - *Low diaphragm*: e.g. due to emphysema
  - *Riedel's lobe*: a non-significant congenital enlargement
- **Malignancy**, e.g.:
  - *Metastases* from a distant carcinoma, particularly bronchus, breast or bowel
  - *Hepatoma*
- **Infection**, e.g.:
  - *Viruses*: viral hepatitis or infectious mononucleosis
  - *Bacteria*: pyogenic abscess

○ *Protozoa*: malaria, kala-azar (leishmaniasis) or amoebic abscess
○ *Hydatid cyst* due to the cestode *Echinococcis granulosis*, the dog tapeworm
● **Congestion**, e.g. right heart failure, cardiac tamponade or hepatic vein thrombosis
● **Early cirrhosis**
● **Obstructive jaundice**
● **Haematological conditions**, e.g. leukaemia, lymphoma or myelofibrosis
● **Infiltration**, most commonly with fat or rarely with amyloid. The four main causes of an enlarged fatty liver are:
○ Obesity
○ Alcohol
○ Starvation
○ Diabetes mellitus

Spleen

● **Lower border:** Start in the left lower quadrant, as the spleen may be unexpectedly large, and work upwards towards the left lower ribs.

● **Upper border:** Start in the chest in the middle of the left anterior axillary line and percuss diagonally across the upper part of the abdomen towards the umbilicus.

● Normally, there is no splenic dullness.

● Dullness over the lower left ribs and/or left side of the upper abdomen suggests an enlarged spleen, the causes of which are listed in Box 10.5.

> Box 10.5: Causes of a large spleen
>
> - **Congestion**, e.g.:
>   - ○ *Portal hypertension* due to cirrhosis of the liver
>   - ○ *Hepatic or portal vein thrombosis*
> - **Haematological conditions**, e.g. leukaemia, lymphoma, myelofibrosis or haemolytic anaemia
> - **Infection**, e.g.:
>   - ○ *Viruses*: viral hepatitis or infectious mononucleosis
>   - ○ *Bacteria*: septicaemia, infective endocarditis, typhoid or brucellosis
>   - ○ *Protozoa*: malaria or kala-azar
> - **Autoimmune diseases (occasionally)**, e.g. rheumatoid arthritis, systemic lupus erythematosus, sarcoidosis or rarely Graves' disease
> - **Storage diseases**, e.g. Gaucher's disease (very rare)

Ascites

- Ascites is defined as fluid in the peritoneal cavity, and may be demonstrated by two tests, namely *shifting dullness* and *fluid thrill.*

Shifting dullness

- Ask the patient to roll over to one side and percuss his abdomen from the dependent side upwards.

- Any fluid that is present will have drained to the dependent side, where percussion will be dull. By contrast, due to the presence of gas-filled bowel floating on top of the fluid, percussion over the elevated side will be resonant.

- Now ask the patient to reverse his position and roll onto his other side. The percussion notes will reverse as any fluid that is present will have moved to the side that was previously uppermost, hence the term 'shifting dullness'.

Fluid thrill

- Ask the patient to place the medial side of either of his hands along the middle of his abdomen, so that it will act as a baffle to prevent vibration being conducted from one side of his abdomen to the other via the abdominal wall.

● Now place the fingers of your *right* hand flat on the left side of the abdomen.

● With the fingers of your *left* hand, flick the right side of the abdominal wall.

● The flick will be felt as a vibration by your right hand only if fluid is present to conduct the vibration.

● The causes of ascites are listed in Box 10.6.

Note!

Shifting dullness is usually more accurate than fluid thrill.

Box 10.6: Causes of ascites

● Most common causes = cirrhosis of the liver, right heart failure, malignant ascites and acute bacterial peritonitis

Mechanisms
● *Portal hypertension*, i.e. increased hydrostatic pressure in the portal vein due to cirrhosis of the liver, right heart failure, constrictive pericarditis, hepatic vein thrombosis (Budd–Chiari syndrome)
● *Malignant invasion* of the peritoneum (malignant ascites)
● *Infection* of the peritoneum, e.g. acute bacterial peritonitis or occasionally tuberculosis
● *Low osmotic pressure* at the venous end of the capillaries due to hypoalbuminaemia, starting in logical order with protein entering the body and finishing with protein loss from the body:
  ○ Malabsorption
  ○ Failure of the liver to manufacture protein

○ Protein-losing enteropathy
○ Nephrotic syndrome
● *Rare causes*
  ○ Triad of ovarian fibroma, ascites and pleural effusion (Meigs' syndrome)
  ○ Hypothyroidism

Palpation

Remember to observe the patient's face for pain as you palpate the abdomen.

Order of palpation
● Light palpation
● Deep palpation
● Liver
● Spleen
● Kidneys
● Aorta
● Bladder/uterus

Light palpation

This is done mainly to detect superficial tenderness.

● Using *the pads* of the fingers of your right hand and *comparing one side with the other*, gently palpate all four quadrants *superficially* for any tenderness, rigidity or masses by making small, slow circular movements with your hand.

● **Rebound tenderness**: If any tenderness is found, test for *rebound tenderness*, a sign of peritoneal inflammation, that is, peritonitis, by observing the patient's face for pain as you quickly remove your hand, causing the peritoneum to rebound quickly. The clinical features of peritonitis are listed in Box 10.7.

> ### Box 10.7: Clinical features of peritonitis
>
> **Symptoms**
> ● Vomiting
> ● Severe abdominal pain
>
> **Signs**
> ● Ill looking; pyrexia
> ● *Localized peritonitis*: localized tenderness ++ and rebound ++ on light palpation
> ● *Generalized peritonitis*: rigid abdomen with generalized tenderness ++ and rebound ++ on light palpation
> ● Bowel sounds absent with generalized disease

Deep palpation

This is carried out mainly to detect masses and organomegaly.

● Using either the right hand alone or the right hand steadied by the left hand placed over its back (Fig. 10.1), make slow circular movements with both *the tips and distal pads* of

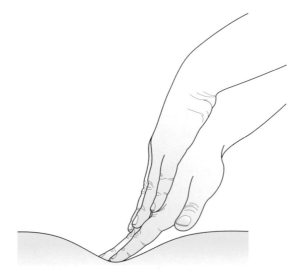

Fig 10.1 Deep palpation, placing the left hand over the back of the right hand

your fingers to palpate all four quadrants *deeply* for deep tenderness, masses and organomegaly, remembering *to compare one side with the other.*

Liver

● Start in the right lower quadrant and work upwards towards the right lower ribs, using either your right hand alone or your right hand steadied by your left hand placed over its back.

● Palpate, that is, gently but firmly push in with the tips and pads of your fingers at the same time as asking the patient to inspire and take a big breath.

Note!

Asking the patient to take a big breath as you push in causes the liver to move down to meet your fingers and increases the likelihood of feeling it. Note that the liver may be just palpable, that is, 'tipped', in a healthy person. The causes of a large liver are listed in Box 10.4 (page 145).

Spleen

● Start in the left lower quadrant and work upwards towards the left lower ribs, using either your right hand alone or your right hand steadied by your left hand placed over its back.

● Palpate, that is, gently but firmly push in with the tips and pads of your fingers at the same time as asking the patient to inspire and take a big breath.

● Normally, the spleen is not palpable. If it is not but you suspect it is enlarged, ask the patient to roll over onto his right side and place your left hand over the back of his left lower ribs. Now palpate in the left upper quadrant by pushing in gently with the tips and pads of the fingers of your right hand at the same time as asking the patient to inspire and take a big breath. In addition, while you are pushing in with your right hand, pull the organ towards your palpating fingers by pulling gently forwards on the back of the patient's ribs with your left hand

- The causes of an enlarged spleen are listed in Box 10.5 (page 147).

- If the spleen is palpable, ask the patient to lie in the supine position and explore its surface and margins for the four clinical signs of an enlarged spleen listed in Box 10.8.

Box 10:8 Four clinical signs of an enlarged spleen

- Dullness to percussion
- You cannot get your fingers above it
- It moves down on respiration
- It has a palpable notch (the hilum) on its medial side

Kidneys

This is performed on both sides with the patient lying supine.

- **Right kidney:** Place the fingers of your *left* hand *pointing medially at right angles to the midline* over the front of the patient's right flank, and the fingers of your right hand *pointing medially at right angles to the midline* behind the patient in the renal triangle on the same side.

- Now 'ballotte' the kidney by gently squeezing and making gentle bouncing movements with the hand at the back, so as to bounce the kidney against the hand on the front.

- Repeat on the left side, but in this case place the fingers of your *right hand pointing laterally* at right angles to the midline on the front of the patient's left flank, and the fingers of your left hand pointing medially behind the patient in his left renal triangle.

● The kidneys may be palpable occasionally in healthy people, particularly on the right side.

> **Note!**
>
> An enlarged kidney feels like a grapefruit, and may be caused by:
> ● polycystic disease
>
> ● tumour (usually a primary tumour).
>
> ● hydronephrosis (rarely palpable).

Aorta

● The aorta is most easily palpated with the tips of the fingers.

● To do this, extend the fingers of both hands and place them *vertically* with the palms and fingers *facing laterally* about 2–3 cm apart over or slightly to the left of the midline at or a little above the umbilicus.

● Gently push in with the tips of the fingers of both hands until you feel a pulsation.

● Determine the width of the pulsation by measuring the distance between the tips of your fingers; it is normally less than 2.5 cm in diameter.

● A pulsatile swelling of over 2.5 cm suggests an aneurysm (that is, an abnormal dilatation of the vessel) and should be investigated by ultrasound.

Bladder and uterus

● If enlargement of the bladder or uterus is suspected, percuss and palpate the area above the pubic symphysis.

Anus and rectum

If you are not later proceeding to examine the genitals as described in Chapter 19, perform a rectal examination at this juncture, as described on page 282, remembering to ignore the reference to the prostate gland when examining a woman.

BACKGROUND INFORMATION

Bowel sounds, renal bruits and other signs in the abdomen

Increased bowel sounds

Increased bowel sounds of a high-pitch tinkling quality are heard in *intestinal obstruction* and are due to increased peristalsis. The causes of intestinal obstruction and the clinical features of its most common cause, carcinoma of the bowel, are listed in Boxes 10.2 and 10.3 (page 144).

Absent bowel sounds

Absent bowel sounds are due to lack of peristalsis (ileus), most commonly in association with inflammation of the bowel resulting from *peritonitis* or ileus in the hours immediately after surgery. An absence of bowel sounds is occasionally due to ileus caused by severe hypokalaemia. The clinical features of peritonitis are listed in Box 10.7 (page 150).

Renal bruits

A bruit due to renal artery stenosis may occasionally be heard in patients with hypertension, but a similar bruit may also be heard in normotensive individuals without renal artery stenosis. A renal bruit is therefore a non-specific sign, although it should be investigated in anyone with hypertension.

Murphy sign

Murphy's sign is a sign of acute cholecystitis and is a temporary arrest of breathing due to pain on deep palpation of the right subcostal area.

McBurney's point

McBurney's point is the junction of the outer and middle thirds of an imaginary line joining the umbilicus to the anterior superior iliac spine, and is approximately over the site of the appendix.

Differential diagnosis of a mass in the left hypochondrium

This is listed in Box 10.9 and is included as it is sometimes a cause of contention among clinicians. The way to think about it is to consider all the organs in the area.

Box 10.9: Differential diagnosis of a mass in the left hypochondrium

- **Enlarged spleen** due to the causes listed in Box 10.5 (page 147)
- **Enlarged left lobe of the liver** due to cancer, abscess or cirrhosis
- **Enlarged splenic flexure of the colon** due to cancer, diverticular abscess or faeces
- **Enlarged left kidney** due to polycystic disease, cancer or hydronephrosis
- **Enlarged stomach** due to cancer or pyloric stenosis
- **Enlarged pancreas** due to cancer or a cyst
- **Retroperitoneal tumour** due to sarcoma (rare)

11

MENTAL STATUS EXAMINATION

EXAMINATION

You should have begun to assess the patient's mental state from
the moment he walked in through the door of your office, or
you approached his bed or entered his home, noting his bearing,
manner, mood and such factors as non-verbal communication,
ranging from his facial expressions to his dress and the state of
his home. In addition, further information should have been
gleaned during the history and physical examination.

The parameters of mental function that should be noted as the
interview proceeds are as follows:

- **Mood/emotional state**: note any anxiety, depression,
  inappropriate euphoria, inappropriate emotional response or
  emotional blunting.

- **Language**: assess the fluency (which is independent of
  content) and comprehension of the spoken word, and the
  ability of the patient to respond to simple requests.

- **Memory**: if you have doubts about the patient's memory,
  test his short-term memory by asking him about
  information given during the interview, and his long-term
  memory by asking him about events in his childhood and

family, such as where he was born and the name of the town in which he lived and went to school.

- **Orientation:** assess orientation by noting if the patient is aware of where he is in both time and place.

- **Thought content:** assess thought content by noting any flights of ideas, obsessions (recurrent thoughts, impulses or images) or compulsions (a need to repeatedly perform a purposeful action).

- **Abnormal beliefs and perceptions:** note any delusions (persistent unshakeable abnormal beliefs), illusions (misinterpretations of external stimuli) or hallucinations (perceptions in the absence of appropriate stimuli).

- **Insight:** assess the patient's insight by noting whether he is aware of the implications of his situation and illness.

- **Abstract thinking:** note whether the patient is able to think in terms of ideas rather than events and things. If necessary, this can be tested by asking simple questions that deal with simple ideas, such as 'What is the similarity between a car and a train?' or 'What is the difference between a ship like the Queen Elizabeth and a submarine?'

Mini Mental Status Examination (MMSE)

If there is any doubt about the patient's state of cognition (i.e. mental processes) and whether or not he is confused/demented, it is appropriate to apply the MMSE, devised by Dr Folstein and colleagues in 1975.

BACKGROUND INFORMATION ABOUT THE MMSE

The MMSE is a quick test that takes between 5 and 10 minutes to administer. It is important to understand that it does not test mood, abnormal forms of thinking or abnormal mental experiences, that is, it is not a test for the diagnosis of anxiety, depression or schizophrenia.

The test consists of two sections. The first section requires verbal answers, tests orientation, attention and memory, and carries a maximum score of 21. The second section tests the ability to name objects, follow verbal and written commands, write a sentence spontaneously and copy a complex polygon diagram, and carries a maximum score of 9. A perfect total score is therefore 30. A score of 24 or above is considered normal. A score of less suggests dementia (or confusion if the condition is reversible).

The test is probably best applied at the end of the history or immediately before the examination of the central nervous system. It may be administered by a doctor, nurse, volunteer or other health worker.

● **Limitations of the MMSE:** The MMSE does not replace clinical assessment in the diagnostic process, but it can contribute to it.

Equipment needed

● Bright lighting
● Copy of the Folstein Mini Mental Status Examination
● Ballpoint pen or pencil and two pieces of paper, one for the patient to fold, the other to be attached to a clipboard on which the patient can write and draw

Position of the patient

● The patient should be seated in quiet, warm surroundings where the test can be carried out without interruption or embarrassment

---

The examination

Table 11.1 shows the MMSE test.

Reference

Folstein MF, Folstein SE, McHugh PR. A practical method for grading the cognitive state of patients for the clinician. *Journal of Psychiatric Research* 1975; 12, 189–198.

Table 11.1 The Mini Mental Status Examination

Date orientation	Tell me the day of the week.....the month..... the year.....the date.....the season of the year	One point for each of the day of the week, the month, the year, the date and the season of the year	5
Place orientation	Which country are you in? Which county? Which town? What is this building? Which floor or room are you in?	One point for each of the country, the county, the town, the building, the floor or room	5
Register 3 objects	Name three objects slowly and clearly, then ask the patient to repeat them	One point for each item correctly repeated	3
Serial sevens	Ask the patient to subtract 7 from 100, and then subtract 7 from the answer, and so on for five answers. Alternatively ask the patient to spell the word 'world' backwards	One point for each correct answer (or letter)	5
Recall 3 objects	Ask the patient to recall the objects mentioned above	One point for each object correctly remembered	3
Naming	Point to your watch and ask the patient 'What is this?' Repeat with a pencil	One point for each correct answer	2
Repeating a phrase	Ask the patient to say, 'No ifs, and no buts'	One point if successful on the first try	1
Verbal commands	Give the patient a piece of plain paper and say, 'Take this paper in your right hand, fold it in half, and put it on the floor'	One point for each correct action	3
Written commands	Show the patient a piece of paper with 'CLOSE YOUR EYES' printed on it	One point if the patient's eyes close	1
Writing	Ask the patient to write a sentence	One point if the sentence has a subject, a verb and makes sense	1

Drawing	Ask the patient to copy a pair of intersecting polygons onto a piece of paper	One point if the drawing has ten corners and two intersecting lines	1
Scoring	A score of 24 or above is considered normal		30

CRANIAL NERVES

EXAMINATION

Cranial nerve I: the olfactory nerve

Sense of smell

- Ask the patient if his sense of smell is intact.

- Test the patency of each side of the nose by asking the patient to block one nostril and breathe in through the other nostril.

● Ask the patient to close his eyes and tell you what he smells as he sniffs at familiar items such as vanilla, gum, coffee, soap, cloves, etc.

> **Note!**
>
> Anosmia (lack of a sense of smell) may be due to a viral infection such as a cold, polyps, drugs (occasionally), trauma to the head or a frontal tumour that has disrupted the fibres of the olfactory nerves.

Eye (cranial nerves II, III, IV and VI)

> So you don't forget any aspect of the examination of the eye, remember that it consists of five parts and that they are usually tested in the following order:
>
> ● visual acuity
> ● visual fields
> ● eye movements
> ● pupils
> ● optic fundus.

Visual acuity (cranial nerve II)

● If required, the patient may wear spectacles for this test, but the fact should be recorded in his notes.

● Use a large Snellen chart at a distance of 6 m (20 feet in the USA) from the patient, or a modified small hand-held chart at the distance indicated on the chart.

● Ask the patient to cover one eye and read the lowest line he can see clearly.

● The visual acuity is the lowest line in which he can read all the letters, although some testers accept the line in which he can read more than half the letters, and record this fact.

● Repeat the test on the other eye.

Note!

Visual acuity is indicated on most charts by the two small numbers at the side of the lowest line in which the patient can read all or more than half the numbers, for example 6/15 (20/50 in the USA). The first number is the distance of the patient from a large Snellen chart; the second number is the distance at which a normal eye can read the line of letters on the same chart. Clearly, the greater the second (or bottom) number, the worse the vision. Normal vision is 6/6 (20/20 in the USA).

Box 12.1: More common causes of a red eye

- Conjunctivitis (infective or allergic)
- Acute closed-angle glaucoma
- Iritis including reactive arthritis (Reiter's syndrome)
- Scleritis/episcleritis
- Subconjunctival haemorrhage, often secondary to trauma or a cough

Visual fields (cranial nerve II)

- Stand about 1 m in front of the patient and ask him to keep his head still and look at your nose without moving his eyes.

Hemianopia and quadrantianopia – peripheral vision tested with both eyes open

- Straighten your arms and hands and place them above and lateral to your shoulders at an angle of 45° to the vertical and half way between you and the patient (Fig. 12.1).

- Now test the vision in the *upper quadrants* of the patient's visual fields (lower retinal quadrants) by asking him to tell you or point each time you randomly tweak one or other of your index fingers.

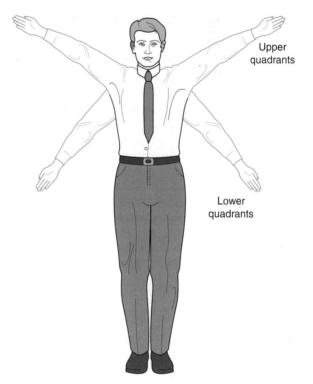

Fig 12.1 Testing the visual fields

- Note any movement the patient fails to see.

- Repeat the procedure for the *lower quadrants* (upper retinal quadrants) with your arms outstretched and abducted laterally at 45° to the sides of your body; again note any movement the patient fails to see.

- Normally, the patient will see each movement of your fingers. Failure to do so in both the upper and lower quadrants on one or both sides of his visual fields suggests a *hemianopia*, or in one quadrant suggests a *quandrantianopia*, both of which involve partial loss of vision in *both* eyes, as demonstrated in Fig. 12.4 (page 176).

Scotoma – partial loss of vision in *one* eye tested on one eye at a time

● While your arms are still in the lower position abducted laterally at 45° to your side, ask the patient to cover one eye with his hand; then close your opposite eye so you can use your own vision as a standard against which to measure the patient's vision.

● Ask the patient to tell you or point each time he sees a finger move as you tweak one or other of your fingers while gradually moving them in to the centre of his visual fields. Note any movement you see but he fails to see.

● Move your arms to their original position above and lateral to your shoulders and repeat the procedure for the upper quadrants. Then repeat the whole procedure on the other eye.

> ### Note!
>
> Background information about the visual fields, hemianopias and scotomata is on page 175.

Eye movements

Cranial nerves III, IV and VI: the oculomotor, trochlear and abducens nerves

● Ask the patient if he experiences any double vision, and then proceed as follows.

● Stand about 1 m in front of the patient and ask him to keep his head still.

● Now place the index finger of your right hand about 30 cm in front of his eyes. Ask him to follow your finger with his eyes and tell you if he experiences any double vision as you move your finger *slowly* in a rectangle measuring about 60 cm across and 50 cm deep (i.e. 25 cm up and 25 cm down from the level of his eyes). Stop for about 2 seconds in the corners of the rectangle and ask about double vision, and for about 5 seconds in the middle of each vertical (i.e. lateral) side of the rectangle and in the middle of the upper horizontal side to check for nystagmus (which, if present, may have a latent period or delay in onset of up to about 5 seconds).

● Finally, test convergence of the eyes by asking the patient to follow your finger as you bring it towards his nose.

Note!

Background information about abnormalities of eye movements and nystagmus is on pages 177–180.

Pupil

Size and regularity

● Inspect the pupils for size and regularity

● They are normally round and equal.

Reaction to light

● **Direct reaction:** Use a torch to test the direct reaction of the pupil to light by shining the light *from the side* into one eye. The pupil of that eye should constrict.

● Repeat on the other eye.

● **Consensual reaction:** Next, test the consensual reaction of the pupil to light by shining the light *from the side* into one eye while watching for constriction of the pupil of the *other* eye.

● Repeat on the other eye.

● **Test for accommodation:** If a consensual reaction does not occur, test the reaction of the pupils to accommodation by placing your right index finger about 10 cm in front of the patient's nose. Now ask the patient to look into the distance. Then ask him to look at your finger, at the same time as checking for constriction of the pupils and convergence of the eyes.

Note!

Background information about the innervation and abnormalities of the pupil is on page 181.

Optic fundus

Visualizing the fundus

- If possible, darken the room in order to dilate the pupil.

- To avoid 'crossing noses', use your right eye to look into the patient's right eye and your left eye to look into the patient's left eye.

- Use the largest round white light produced by the ophthalmoscope and place your index finger on the focusing wheel, that is, the lens disc.

- When looking into the patient's eye, *keep your eye, the aperture of the instrument, the line of light and the patient's pupil in a single straight line, and search for the back of the eye.*

- **Finding the retina**: While you are learning to look into the eye, you may find it helpful to start by looking through the instrument from an angle of about 20° to the temporal side of the midline at a distance of about 60 cm from the patient. Look for the *red reflex*, which is caused by light reflected back from the retina, and then slowly advance towards the patient, keeping the red reflex in your vision all the time.

● **Focusing the instrument**: The focusing wheel or lens disc allows you to compensate for long (far) and short (near) sight and also to look at structures such as the lens. If the retina is blurred due to the patient having long sight, compensate by turning the wheel in a clockwise direction to the plus or green dioptres until the image comes into focus. If the patient is short-sighted, turn the wheel in an anticlockwise direction to the minus or red dioptres.

> ### Note!
>
> The dioptre is the unit used for measuring the power of a lens and is the reciprocal of its focal length measured in metres.

● As soon as you see individual structures *use the following checklist* to look for:
  ○ arteries and veins
  ○ optic disc and cup
  ○ retina
  ○ macula.

Arteries and veins

● Four main sets of arteries and veins radiate out from the optic disc in the following directions: obliquely up to the right on the patient in a 'north-westerly' direction, obliquely up to the left in a 'north-easterly' direction, obliquely down to the left in a 'south-easterly' direction, and obliquely down to the right in a 'south-westerly' direction. The veins are recognized by the fact that they are darker and usually a little plumper than the arteries.

For the *arteries*, look for the following:

● **Tortuosity** due to the blood pressure continually pounding the arteries over many years, causing them to elongate, with the result that they become tortuous, as they have to occupy the same space on the retina as they did when they were shorter.

● **Narrowing** due to spasm of the muscle in the arterial wall.

● **Silver wiring**: a white appearance of the arteries due to light being reflected back from a thickened atherosclerotic arterial wall.

For the *veins*, look for the following:

● Look for arteriovenous nipping due to elongated arteries adopting a twisted position that causes them to lie on the veins, compressing and 'nipping' them (Fig. 12.2).

> ### Note!
>
> Arterial narrowing, tortuosity, arteriovenous nipping and silver wiring are each suggestive of hypertension in persons aged under 60 years, but they also occur with diabetes mellitus and in the elderly with a normal blood pressure.

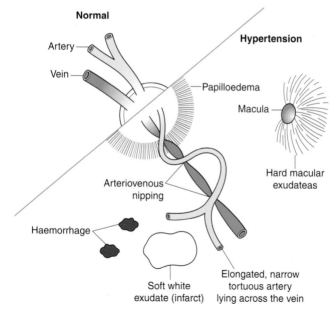

Fig 12.2 Retinopathy

Optic disc

● Find the optic disc by following an artery and vein until you see the demarcated pale, round shape of the disc.

● Having found the disc, look at it carefully for *papilloedema, papillitis, optic atrophy* and *an enlarged optic cup.*

Note!

Background information about abnormalities of the optic fundus is on page 182.

Cranial nerve V: the trigeminal nerve

Cranial nerve V supplies sensory fibres to the skin of the face and the tongue, and motor fibres to the muscles of mastication. These functions are tested as follows.

Motor

● Place the pads of your fingers over the temporal area on either side of the patient's forehead.

● Now ask the patient to clench his teeth at the same time as you palpate and check the strength of contraction of, first, the temporal muscles on either side of the forehead, and then the masseter muscles on either side of the face.

Jaw jerk

● Ask the patient to open his mouth and *relax* his jaw.

● Now place your left index finger horizontally on the relaxed lower jaw beneath the lower lip and gently strike *vertically down* on it with the head of a reflex hammer. A reflex contraction may be seen or felt in some normal people and in upper motor neurone (UMN) lesions.

Sensory

- Advise the patient that you are going to touch his face with the point of a pin or safety-pin and cotton wool, but that you will not hurt him.

- Ask him to close his eyes while you test the ophthalmic, maxillary and mandibular divisions of cranial nerve V on *the forehead, over the maxilla and along the lower jaw.*

- Test each division by gently touching *first one side of the face and then the other* with the point of the pin or safety-pin to test pain sensation, and with the cotton wool to test *light touch.*

- The best technique is to lightly touch each site two or three times in quick succession, so that the patient has a good chance of recognizing the stimulus. As you touch each site, ask the patient what he feels.

- Also test the *corneal reflex* by asking the patient to look to the side while you gently touch his cornea with a piece of cotton wool shaped to a point. The patient will normally blink, but not if the reflex arc has been disrupted, as for example occurs in *brainstem death.*

- Sensation of the tongue is not normally tested.

Cranial nerve VII: the facial nerve

The facial nerve supplies motor fibres to the muscles of the face for both voluntary and emotional movements, and sensory fibres to the taste buds on the anterior two-thirds of the tongue. It also sends a branch to the stapedius muscle in the ear. However, only motor function to the face is usually tested.

- Test the nerve by asking the patient to perform the following movements, one after the other: close his eyes tightly, show you his teeth, smile, blow out his cheeks, look up and wrinkle his forehead.

> ## Note!
>
> Background information about abnormalities of cranial nerve VII is on page 186.

Cranial nerve VIII: the acoustic nerve

Cranial nerve VIII supplies sensory nerves that run centrally from the inner ear (i.e. from the cochlea and vestibular apparatus) to the brainstem and are involved in hearing and balance.

Tests of cranial nerve VIII and its connections

- Normally only hearing is tested.

- Ask the patient whether he has a hearing problem.

- Test the hearing of each ear in turn by pressing on the tragus of one ear and then asking the patient to repeat what you say as you whisper softly into the other ear from a distance of about 15–20 cm.

Weber's and Rinne's tests

These tests can be used to differentiate between conduction and nerve deafness.

- First set the tuning fork vibrating by striking it on a solid object such a table.

Weber's test: Place the vibrating tuning fork on the middle of the scalp or on the middle of the forehead and ask the patient where he perceives the vibration.

Rinne's test: Place the vibrating tuning fork on the mastoid process. Ask the patient when he no longer hears or feels the vibration, and when that occurs, move the fork (which should still be vibrating) to the air beside the ear and ask the patient if he can still hear it.

- Repeat on the other side.

> # Note!
>
> Background information about cranial nerve VIII, Weber's and Rinne's tests is on page 187.

Cranial nerves IX and X: the glossopharyngeal and vagus nerves

Cranial nerves IX and X supply both motor and sensory fibres to the pharynx. In addition, cranial nerve IX also supplies sensory fibres for taste to the posterior one third of the tongue, and cranial nerve X supplies motor fibres to the palate and parasympathetic fibres to the viscera of the thorax and abdomen.

● Note any nasal quality or slurring of the patient's voice due to weakness of the pharyngeal muscles. Such a speech defect is known as *dysarthria* and is discussed on page 192.

Motor function

● Ask the patient to open his mouth and say 'Ah' as you observe his uvula. If necessary, use a torch or light to illuminate the mouth and a spatula to depress the tongue. Movement of the uvula is normally symmetrically upwards, or *away from* the side of any weakness, as the muscles on the normal side contract and pull the uvula towards them.

Sensory function

● Advise the patient what you intend to do and, if he agrees, ask him to open his mouth wide. Now evoke the gag reflex by touching the back of his pharynx with a tongue depressor or a Q-tip. Failure to gag suggests either sensory or motor loss to the pharynx.

> ## Note!
>
> Malfunction of these nerves may be caused by conditions such as:
>
> - strokes involving the brainstem
> - pharyngeal cancer invading the nerves
> - denervation of the motor nerves due to motor neurone disease.

Cranial nerve XI: the spinal accessory nerve

This nerve is solely motor and supplies only the trapezius and sternomastoid muscles.

- *Trapezius muscles* are tested by asking the patient to shrug both his shoulders and maintain them in the shrugged position while you try to push each of them down.

- *Sternomastoid muscles* are tested one at a time by asking the patient to turn his head to the side while you oppose him by pressing against his lower jaw with the pads of the fingers of one of your hands. Because of the way the muscle is inserted into the back of the skull, this tests the sternomastoid muscle of the side opposite to the direction in which the head is turned, as illustrated in Fig. 12.3.

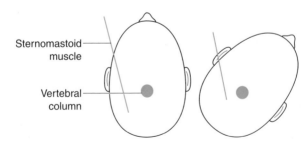

Fig 12.3 Contraction of the sternomastoid muscle causing the head to rotate to the opposite side

Cranial nerve XII: the hypoglossal nerve

This nerve is solely motor and supplies only the tongue.

● Cranial nerve XII is tested by asking the patient to protrude his tongue straight out and then waggle it about as quickly as possible while you look for asymmetry of its shape or movements.

Note!

Background information about abnormalities of cranial nerve XII is on page 189.

BACKGROUND INFORMATION

Visual fields

The most common visual field defects are hemianopia and scotoma, both of which are described below. The pathways associated with these defects are illustrated in Fig. 12.4, which also shows a quick way of drawing and remembering the optic pathways.

Homonymous hemianopia

This type of hemianopia involves a loss of vision on one side of the visual field, that is, on the temporal side of one eye and the nasal side of the other eye, and is due to a lesion in the posterior part of the cerebral cortex lobe on the side opposite to the loss of vision (Fig. 12.4C).

The most common cause of homonymous hemianopia is a stroke. If the stroke (or other lesion affecting the cortex) is large, it may involve the motor and/or sensory cortex, which also serves the opposite side of the body. Thus, the defect in the visual field associated with a homonymous hemianopia is always on the *same* side as any hemiparesis.

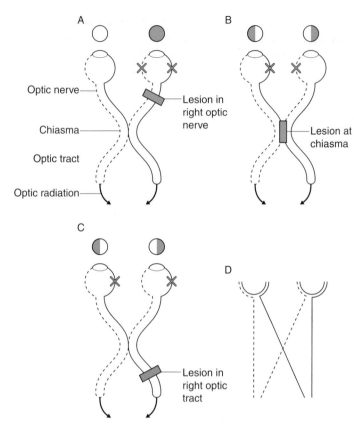

Fig 12.4 Visual field defects. (A) Blind right eye. (B) Bitemporal hemianopia. (C) Left homonymous hemianopia. (D) Quick way of drawing and remembering the visual fields and pathways

Bitemporal hemianopia

This type of hemianopia involves a loss of the outer half of the visual fields on both sides due to a lesion such as a pituitary tumour compressing the central fibres of the optic chiasma. As a result, the nerve fibres supplying the nasal side of both retinas no longer function normally, and the patient is unable to see to the side, although he can still see to the front as the nerve fibres supplying the temporal sides of the retinas are still functioning (Fig. 12.4B).

Typically, bitemporal hemianopia results in the patient bumping into things and not being able to see the end of a line of type or writing when he is reading. Bitemporal hemianopia is much less common than homonymous hemianopia.

Scotoma

This involves a loss of part of the vision in one eye as a result of a lesion in the *retina* or *optic nerve* rather than the chiasma or cerebral cortex. Scotomas (other than the naturally occurring blind spot) are caused by conditions such as:

- localized detachment of the retina

- lesions that affect only part of the cross-section of the optic nerve, such as the demyelination associated with multiple sclerosis

- damage to localized areas of the retina, such as occurs with infection due to toxoplasmosis.

Cranial nerves III, IV and VI and nystagmus

Cranial nerve III supplies the superior, inferior and medial rectus muscles as well as the inferior oblique muscle. Cranial nerve IV supplies the superior oblique muscle, and Cranial nerve VI the lateral rectus muscle.

Eye movements are under the control of both UMNs and lower motor neurones (LMNs) and their connections. The UMNs, that is, cells in the cerebral cortex and their axons, control *conjugate* movements of the eyes, meaning that they ensure that when the eyes move, they both move together. Lesions of these nerves (most commonly due to strokes) therefore result in conjugate defects of eye movements, meaning that both eyes are deviated equally to one side or the other, so double vision (i.e. diplopia) does not occur.

The LMNs, meaning the nuclei and nerve fibres of cranial nerves III, IV and VI and certain of their connections, as demonstrated in Fig. 12.5, control the movements of each eye independently.

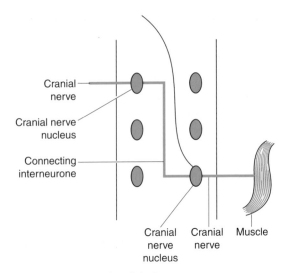

Fig 12.5 Sites of lesions causing diplopia

Lesions of the LMNs therefore result in paresis of a single eye and so cause misalignment of the eyes and double vision. Of the lesions affecting these nerves, those of cranial nerve VI are the most common, due, it is said, to its long intracranial course.

In summary:

● Conjugate defect = upper motor neurone lesion.

● Diplopia = lower motor neurone, interneurone or muscular lesion.

Clinical features of lesions of cranial nerves III, IV and VI

As mentioned above, a lesion at any of the sites labelled in Fig. 12.5 results in misalignment of the eyes and double vision, that is, diplopia. The other manifestations of lesions affecting cranial nerves III, IV and VI are as follows.

Cranial nerve III (superior, inferior and medial rectus muscles plus the inferior oblique muscle)

● **Ptosis** (drooping of the upper eyelid) as the upper eyelid is innervated by cranial nerve III, as well as by the sympathetic nervous system. The ptosis is sometimes so severe that the eye is completely closed.

- **Downward and outward deviation of the eye**: this is due to the unopposed actions of the muscles innervated by cranial nerves IV and VI. It is sometimes necessary to lift the eyelid in order to demonstrate this.

- **Pupil dilation**: this is due to the lesion affecting the parasympathetic nerves running to the pupil via cranial nerve III causing paresis of the constrictor muscle of the pupil.

Remember that the eye is 'down and out' with a lesion due to cranial nerve III.

Weber's syndrome is palsy of cranial nerve III plus hemiparesis on the opposite side of the body, and is due to ischaemic damage of both the nucleus of cranial nerve III and the nearby corticospinal tract supplying the limbs on the opposite side.

Cranial nerve IV (superior oblique muscle)

A lesion of cranial nerve IV may be difficult to detect, as usually there is little misalignment of the eyes. However, looking down and inwards may be difficult and produce visible misalignment and double vision.

Cranial nerve VI (lateral rectus muscle)

The resting position of the eye with a lesion of this nerve is either deceptively normal or deviated medially. The problem is that the eye cannot be moved laterally, and as a result double vision occurs when the patient tries to move his eyes to the side of the lesion, as the unaffected eye moves normally while the affected eye remains stationary. Lesions of cranial nerve VI may be caused by conditions such as diabetes mellitus and raised intracranial pressure.

Nystagmus

Nystagmus is involuntary oscillatory movements of the eyes and may be in a horizontal, vertical or rotatory direction. Nystagmus is most commonly due to lesions in the cerebellum, the vestibular apparatus, the brainstem or the connections between them. It may, however, also be congenital, or acquired from occupations such as mining that are performed in poor light, and may be caused by anti-epileptic drugs such as phenytoin, phenobarbitone and diazepam.

The fast phase is the active movement of the phenomenon, and the slow phase is the recovery movement. In cerebellar disease, nystagmus is often demonstrable when the patient looks towards the side of the lesion.

Box 12.2 contains information about brainstem strokes, diplopia and other cranial nerve palsies.

Box 12.2: Cranial nerve palsies and the clinical features of brainstem infarction (i.e. brainstem stroke)

- Various syndromes and patterns of symptoms and signs that include:
- **Coma** if the brainstem reticular formation is involved
- **Nausea, vomiting**
- **Combinations of cranial nerve palsies** that include vertigo (cranial nerve VIII), double vision (cranial nerves III, IV and VI), ipsilateral facial pain and numbness (cranial nerve V), ipsilateral facial palsy (cranial nerve VII), tinnitus and ipsilateral deafness (cranial nerve VIII), nystagmus, dysarthria and dysphagia (cranial nerves IX, X and XII)
- **Ipsilateral cerebellar ataxia**
- **Contralateral loss of pain and temperature sensation** due to involvement of the lateral spinothalamic tract
- **Contralateral hemiplegia** due to involvement of the corticospinal tract
- **Conjugate lateral gaze palsy**: inability to move the eyes to the side

- **Locked-in syndrome**, which is due to a lesion in the ventral pons severing the connections between the cerebral cortex and most of the brainstem. As a result, the patient is conscious with a functioning cerebral cortex, but is 'locked in' and unable to speak, move or communicate except by eye movements

Pupil

The pupil is innervated by parasympathetic nerves running with cranial nerve III that supply its *circular constrictor* muscle fibres, and also by sympathetic nerves that run along the carotid artery and supply its *radial dilator* muscle fibres.

Argyll Robertson pupil

This is a small irregular unreactive pupil that occurs in tertiary syphilis.

Iritis

Iritis may result in adhesions between the iris and the lens and so cause an irregular unreactive pupil.

Opiate drugs

These cause a small constricted unreactive pupil.

Holmes–Adie pupil

Holmes–Adie pupil is a dilated unreactive or almost unreactive pupil usually associated with absent tendon reflexes that is seen mainly in young women, in whom it may be of sudden onset and associated with blurred vision. It is due to degeneration of the postganglionic parasympathetic nerve fibres running to the pupil.

Horner's syndrome

Horner's syndrome is a constellation of signs that are due to dysfunction of the sympathetic nerves to the orbit and face, most commonly as a result of infiltration of the stellate ganglion by an apical carcinoma of the bronchus.

Clinically, Horner's syndrome consists of the following four features:

- ptosis – drooping of the upper eyelid

- myosis – small pupil

- anhydrosis – lack of sweating on the affected side

- enophthalmus – sunken eye (the least common sign).

Optic fundus

Papilloedema

Papilloedema is oedema of the optic nerve at the point at which it enters the eye, and is recognized by loss of definition, swelling and blurring of the border of the disc accompanied by distension of the retinal veins. Papilloedema is caused by raised intracranial pressure and malignant hypertension.

Optic atrophy

Optic atrophy is the result of the death of axons in the retina and optic nerve and *is recognized by a pathologically white or whitish-grey appearance* of the optic disc. According to its appearance on fundoscopy, optic atrophy is classified into two types: primary and secondary.

Primary optic atrophy

In this condition, *there is no preceding swelling of the disc*, and as a consequence *the white margin of the disc is very clearly demarcated* from the surrounding pink of the retina. Primary optic atrophy may be caused by:

- pressure on the optic nerve by tumours

- deficiency of vitamin B_{12} or thiamine

- hereditary conditions such as Leber's disease

● toxicity due to heavy metals and drugs such as chloroquine and several anti-tuberculous drugs.

Secondary optic atrophy

In this condition, *there is preceding swelling of the disc followed by gliosis.* As a consequence, *the disc is pale but its margin is blurred and not very well demarcated.* Secondary optic atrophy may result from chronic papilloedema and papillitis (which is inflammation and increased vascularity causing swelling of the optic nerve where it enters the eye, due, for instance, to acute demyelination associated with multiple sclerosis; Box 12:3).

Box 12.3: Clinical features of multiple sclerosis

A disease involving areas of demyelination of nerves + axon damage, mainly in the white matter but also the grey matter of the central nervous system. Clinically multiple sclerosis usually presents in one of two ways:
● **Pattern 1** (85% of cases): *Relapsing and remitting* disease with sudden onset of symptoms and signs that affect different parts of the body at different times causing any of the following:
● *Optic nerve demyelination* (optic neuritis), resulting in blurring or loss of vision that is often only temporary
● *Brainstem demyelination* affecting the cranial nerves and causing double vision, vertigo, facial numbness/weakness and/or dysphagia
● *Spinal cord demyelination* causing sudden onset of numbness or weakness of a leg with dragging of the foot, or spastic paraplegia with upper motor neurone signs (see page 212). Note: This pattern of disease is sometimes associated with an electric sensation passing down the trunk and the limbs when the patient bends his neck or coughs (Lhermitte's sign)
● **Pattern 2**: (15% of cases): *Primary progressive* disease with a slow unremitting pattern that may result in chronic spastic paraplegia with upper motor neurone signs (see page 212)

Enlargement of the optic cup

The peripheral part of the optic disc is largely made up of nerve fibres. The central part or *optic cup* is paler and does not contain nerve fibres but is where blood vessels enter and leave the eye. Enlargement of the cup is a sign of glaucoma and is due to the increased intraocular hydrostatic pressure associated with the condition damaging and reducing the number of nerve fibres running through the disc.

Retina

Among the many abnormalities that might be seen in the retina, some of the most common, such as microaneurysms, exudates, haemorrhages and cotton spots are due to *microvascular disease*. Details of these lesions are as follows:

- **Microaneurysms.** Microaneurysms are aneurysmal dilatations of the weakened wall of small blood vessels. On the retina, microaneurysms appear as small red spots about the size of a pinhead; they are seen in diabetes mellitus but not in hypertension.

- **Haemorrhages, exudates and cotton spots.** These are due to particular manifestations of microvascular disease, *are commonly seen in diabetes mellitus, and are the defining sign of malignant hypertension, which, however, is rare.*

The mechanisms by which microvascular disease causes its effects on the retina are twofold, namely *leaks from* and *ischaemia of* small blood vessels.

Leaks from small blood vessels

Leaks of blood result in retinal haemorrhages, leaks of fluid plus protein result in exudates, and leaks of fluid result in oedema, usually around the macula.

- **Haemorrhages** vary in size and are easily recognized as red lesions. Haemorrhages that are deep in the retina appear as either small red *dots* or larger *blots*. Superficial haemorrhages fan out along bundles of nerves to form what are known as *flame haemorrhages.*

- **Proteinous exudates** typically appear as small, yellow, waxy nodules on the retina in diabetes mellitus.

- **Macular oedema** is due to leakage of fluid from small blood vessels and is discussed below under the heading 'Macula'.

Ischaemia of small blood vessels

Ischaemia results in the death of nerve cells, the debris of which is known as *cotton spots.* In addition, ischaemia may also result in *new vessel formation.*

Clinically, cotton spots are recognized as small white patches that look like small pieces of cotton wool against the pink of the retina.

New vessel formation is leashes of small fragile new vessels that are formed in response to ischaemia and originate most commonly at the bifurcation of veins or the point at which veins enter the retina. New vessel formation occurs in diabetes mellitus but not in hypertension. As they are fragile, new vessels have a propensity to bleed and are therefore an indication for urgent treatment.

The top half of Fig. 12.2 (page 169) above represents a normal fundus. The bottom half is a representation of tortuous arteries, arteriovenous nipping, papilloedema, exudates and haemorrhages.

Other pathologies of the retina

Less common lesions of the retina include white denuded areas of retinal destruction due to infections such as toxoplasmosis, and the black lesions of retinitis pigmentosa that are due to proliferation of pigment containing cells and look as if spots of Indian ink have been splattered across the surface of the retina.

Macula

The macular is most easily visualized by asking the patient to look directly into the light of the ophthalmoscope. Among the abnormalities affecting central vision that may be seen in the vicinity of the macular are *macula oedema* and *macular degeneration.*

Macular oedema

Macular oedema is due to fluid leaking as a result of microvascular disease, most commonly in association with diabetes mellitus. Clinically, macular oedema may be visible as obvious swelling of the retina around the macular. However, despite severe oedema, the area around the macular may appear deceptively normal. Because it threatens central vision, macular oedema is an indication for urgent investigation and treatment.

Macular degeneration

The most common form of macular degeneration is the 'dry' form, which is often visible as discrete yellow lesions around the macula. The 'wet' form is less common and is sometimes recognized by a greyish-green colouration due to bleeding between layers of the retina.

> How to differentiate between the retinal changes of diabetes mellitus and malignant hypertension: haemorrhages, exudates and cotton spots occur in both diabetes mellitus, which is common, and malignant hypertension, which is rare. Microaneurysms and new vessels are characteristic of diabetes mellitus but not of malignant hypertension, whereas papilloedema is seen in malignant hypertension but not diabetes mellitus.

Cranial nerve VII

Differentiating between an UMN and a LMN lesion of cranial nerve VII

UMN lesion

The forehead uniquely receives UMNs from *both* sides of the cerebral cortex, whereas *the lower part of the face*, like every other part of the body, receives UMN innervation from *one* side only, that is, from the opposite side. The result is that an *UMN* lesion of cranial nerve VII paralyses only the *lower* part of the face, as the forehead is spared because only one of its two UMNs is affected, as shown in Fig. 12.6. Thus, with an UMN lesion of cranial nerve VII, the patient can still move and wrinkle his forehead, but he cannot move the affected side of his lower face.

Note!

Voluntary and emotional movements of the face are controlled by different UMNs. As a result, *emotional movements* of the face are often *less* affected by an UMN lesion of cranial nerve VII than voluntary movements.

LMN lesion

As illustrated in Fig. 12.6, the LMNs of cranial nerve VII supply *both the upper and lower* parts of the face. The whole side of the face is therefore paralysed by a LMN lesion of cranial nerve VII; that is, both the forehead and the lower part of the face are paralysed.

Bell's palsy is the most common lesion affecting the LMNs to the face. This is due to viral infection of the nerve, usually with herpes simplex virus, although occasionally the causative organism may be the herpes zoster virus, resulting in a condition known as the *Ramsay Hunt syndrome*, in which, due to shingles, the patient experiences paralysis of one side of the face as well as pain and vesicles over the external auditory meatus and the tonsillar fauces.

Weber's and Rinne's tests

Weber's test

Normally, the vibration is heard in the middle of the head.

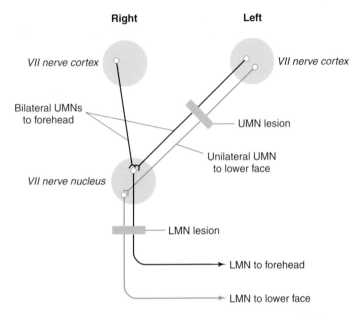

Fig 12.6 Cranial nerve VII lesions. LMN, lower motor neurone; UMN, upper motor neurone

With conduction deafness, the vibration is heard on the *same* side as the deafness, as conduction through bone to the cochlea of that ear is better than conduction through air or bone to the opposite ear. Test this on yourself by performing the test with one ear plugged with a finger.

Conversely, with nerve deafness, the vibration is heard on the side *opposite* to the deafness, as the nerve-deaf ear is neurologically 'dead' and the vibration can only be perceived by the normal ear.

Rinne's test

Normally, the vibration can still be heard when the tuning fork is moved to the side of the ear, as air conduction is normally better than bone conduction.

With conduction deafness, the vibration is loudest when the tuning fork is placed on the mastoid process on the *same* side as the deafness, as conduction through bone to the cochlea of that ear is better than conduction through air or bone to the opposite ear. Test this on yourself by performing the test with one ear plugged with a finger.

Conversely, with nerve deafness, the vibration is heard in the ear *opposite* to the deaf ear when the tuning fork is placed on the mastoid process of the deaf ear, as that ear is neurologically 'dead,' and the vibration can only be perceived by the normal ear.

Cranial nerve XII

Normally, the tongue protrudes straight out.

LMN lesion

As with any other LMN lesion, the weakness is on the same side as the lesion, with the result that the normal or strong side of the tongue *pushes the tongue towards the side of the lesion*, or alternatively protrudes it straight out if the lesion and the weakness are bilateral.

UMN lesion

As with any other UMN lesion, the weakness is on the side opposite to the lesion, with the result that the normal or strong side of the tongue *pushes the tongue to the opposite side to the lesion*.

Weakness of tongue movements may result in slurred speech (i.e. dysarthria), which is discussed on page 192.

Differentiating between an UMN and a LMN lesion of cranial nerve XII

Apart from moving towards the same side as a LMN lesion and the opposite side to an UMN lesion, the appearance of the tongue is also different with the two lesions:

● With an **UMN lesion**, the tongue is spastic and clumsy but looks normal without any wasting or fasciculation.

● With a **LMN lesion,** the tongue is spastic and clumsy, but in addition is also *wasted* and exhibits *fasciculation* on the affected side or on both sides if the lesion and weakness are bilateral.

Note!

Fasciculation is a sign of denervation and a LMN lesion, and is visible as worm-like movements of the epithelium of the tongue (or skin in the case of a muscle other than the tongue). Fasciculation is due to uncoordinated random contractions of individual motor units, each of which consists of a nerve fibre serving a number of muscle fibres.

UMN and LMN lesions of cranial nerve XII may be caused by conditions such as:

● strokes affecting the cerebral cortex or brainstem

● motor neurone disease.

Common speech defects

Dysphasia

Dysphasia is most easily defined as *a thinking or cortical difficulty* with speech. Two main types of dysphasia are recognized.

Broca's dysphasia

Broca's dysphasia (also known as motor or executive dysphasia) is a problem with speech in which the patient has lost fluency but not comprehension, so *knows what he wants to say but cannot say it.*

An easy way to remember the site of the lesion associated with Broca's dysphasia is to remember that a problem of this type is a *motor* problem and that the organs we use for speaking are our lips, tongue, mouth, pharynx and larynx. From this, you might expect that the lesion is in the motor cortex serving these organs. However, it is not quite in these areas, as patients with this type of dysphasia are often still able to move these tissues for voluntary tasks other than speech. Instead, as shown in Fig. 12.7, the lesion is in the cortex *close by* – on the left side *immediately in front* of the motor areas serving the lips, tongue, mouth, pharynx and larynx, that is, in the inferior frontal gyrus known as Broca's area.

Wernicke's dysphasia

Wernicke's dysphasia (also known as sensory or receptive dysphasia) is a much more profound difficulty with speech than Broca's dysphasia, and is loss of the central organization and comprehension of speech. As a result, although the patient can speak, he has lost the ability to understand the spoken or written word, and the content of what he says is an unintelligible mixture of words strung together in what is sometimes known as *jargon aphasia.*

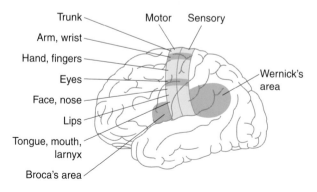

Fig 12.7 Diagrammatic representation of the speech centres

As with Broca's dysphasia, an easy way to remember the site of the lesion associated with Wernicke's dysphasia is to remember that a speech problem of this type is a *sensory* or *receptive* problem, and that the organs we speak with are our lips, tongue, mouth, pharynx and larynx. From this, you might expect the lesion to be in the sensory cortex serving these organs. However, it is not quite in these areas, as patients with this type of dysphasia often still have sensation in these tissues. Instead, as shown in Fig. 12.7, the lesion is in the cortex *close by* – on the left side *immediately behind* the sensory cortex serving the lips, tongue, mouth, pharynx and larynx, that is in the parietotemporal area known as Wernicke's area.

Dysarthria

Dysarthria is defined as *a mechanical difficulty* affecting *the muscles* concerned with speech. Examples of lesions causing dysarthria are lesions of cranial nerves IX, X and XII, and lesions of the cerebellum, in which words are often slurred into one another in what is known as *scanning speech*.

Dysphonia

Dysphonia is defined as difficulty with speech due a lesion affecting *the larynx or its nerve supply.* Dysphonia results in a hoarse or weak voice. Causes of dysphonia include laryngitis, carcinoma of the larynx and lesions of the recurrent laryngeal nerve, most commonly as a result of carcinoma of the bronchus involving the hilum of the left lung or damage occurring during surgery on the thyroid gland.

Stutter and stammer

Stammer and stutter are disorders of articulation affecting the *rhythm* of speech. Their cause is unknown at the present time. *Stutter* involves a gap or halt in the speech; *stammer* involves speaking in a halting *repetitive* manner, for example, 'In-In-In Instead of studying, I-I-I would like-like-like to go-go-go-to the cinema tonight...'.

13

MOTOR SYSTEM

Equipment needed

● Reflex hammer

Position of the patient

● The patient should be sitting or standing in warm, quiet surroundings during examination of the arms, and either lying supine or sitting with his legs dangling during examination of the legs

Order of the examination

● Inspection
● Palpation
● Tone
● Power
● Coordination
● Reflexes

EXAMINATION

Inspection

General inspection (relevant to the motor system)

● Notice the patient's posture, gait, the way he moves and any involuntary movements. Examples of abnormal gaits are on page 39.

Inspection of the arms and legs

● Look for wasting and fasciculation (see page 190) of the muscles in both arms, starting with the muscles around the scapula, then the front and back of the upper arm, and then the muscles of the forearm, thenar and hypothenar eminences and the interosseus muscles.

● Look for wasting and fasciculation of the muscles in the buttocks, thighs and calves of both legs.

Palpation

● Use the fingers and thumbs of both hands to palpate the muscles of the arms and legs on both sides simultaneously, starting with the muscles around the scapulae and shoulders, then the upper and lower arms and the hands, and finally the buttocks, thighs and calves, feeling for their quality and texture and whether there is any wasting.

Muscle tone

Arms

This is performed first on one arm and then the other.

● Ask the patient to sit with an elbow flexed to 90° and relax his arm 'like a jelly'. Then take hold of the arm by the hand and perform at least two of the following tests to assess its tone by:
  ○ extending and flexing the elbow

○ rotating the whole distal part of the limb in a circular
   fashion from the elbow down
○ supination/pronation of the relaxed forearm.
○ release the patient's hand, and ask him to flex his elbow
   and place his forearm in the vertical position with the
   hand at the top. Now take hold of the distal part of his
   forearm and ask him to let his hand go floppy while you
   shake it backwards and forwards in order to assess the
   tone of the muscles supporting the wrist and hand.

Legs

This is performed first on one leg and then the other.

● Ask the patient to relax one of his legs 'like a jelly', and
   then take hold of it above the ankle and assess its tone by:
   ○ extending and flexing the hip and knee
   ○ rotating the whole distal part of the limb in a circular
      fashion.

Note!

● **Increased muscle tone**: Due to imbalance between the
   agonist and antagonist muscles, increased muscle tone is
   found in upper motor neurone (UMN) lesions and
   Parkinson's disease.
● **Decreased muscle tone** is difficult to differentiate from
   normal, but is found in lower motor neurone (LMN) lesions,
   in cerebellar disease and immediately after a stroke (Box
   13.1) or a cord lesion.

Box 13:1: Clinical features of a cerebral hemisphere stroke

Symptoms
- Sudden onset of any or all of the following:
  - ○ Difficulty walking and moving the limbs on one side of the body (hemiplegia)
  - ○ Difficulty speaking (dysphasia; page 190)
  - ○ Loss of vision on one side (homonymous hemianopia; page 175)
- Difficulty swallowing (dysphagia)

Signs
- Weakness of the arm and leg on one side of the body of an upper motor neurone type (page 212), although there may initially be hypotonia and hyporeflexia
- Weakness of the facial muscles of an upper motor neurone type (page 186)
- Loss of sensation on the affected side of the body, possibly only demonstrable by testing for *extinction* (page 219)
- Deviation of the eyes ± the head due to an upper motor neurone lesion affecting conjugate vision (page 177)
- Loss of vision on one side due to homonymous hemianopia Dysphasia (see above)
- Dysphagia

Power

Note!

Inform the patient that the following tests involve seeing how strong he is. It may help if you demonstrate each movement you want the patient to make by doing it yourself as you ask him to do it. Start proximally in the arms by testing the power of the muscles of the shoulders and work distally; then repeat the same sequence in the legs, starting proximally with the muscles of the hips. Weakness of a muscle may be due to an UMN or LMN lesion, or to pain from a lesion in a muscle, bone, tendon, joint or bursa.

Muscles of the arms

Shoulders

Test both sides simultaneously.

- **Abduction** (0–15°: supraspinatus): ask the patient to bend his elbows to about 90° with his arms by his sides.

- Now place your hands on his upper arms immediately above his elbows and ask him to push both arms out to the side (abduction) while you try to stop him by pushing in.

- **Abduction** (15–90°: deltoid): ask the patient to lift his arm laterally (abduction) to shoulder level (Fig. 13.1).

- Now place your hands on his upper arms immediately above his elbows and ask him to stop you while you try to push his arms down.

- **Adduction** (pectoralis major, latissimus dorsi, teres major): ask the patient to lower his arms until they are abducted at about 45° or 50°.

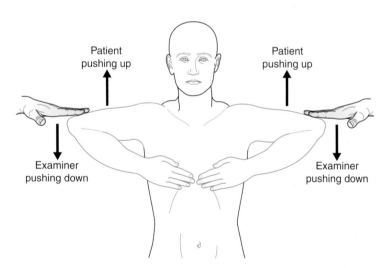

Patient
pushing up

Patient
pushing up

Examiner
pushing down

Examiner
pushing down

Fig 13.1 Testing the power of abduction of the arms

● Now place your hands *under* his elbows and ask him to pull his arms in towards the sides of his trunk while you try to resist him.

Elbows

Test both flexion and extension on one arm, and then repeat on the other arm.

● **Flexion** (biceps, brachialis, brachioradialis): ask the patient to bend both elbows to about 120° with his arms by his sides and his forearms and hands straight out in front of him.

● Now place your hand on the front of his forearm immediately proximal to the wrist and ask him to bend his arm further towards his shoulder while you try to straighten it.

● **Extension** (triceps, anconeus): while the patient's elbows are still flexed to about 120° with his arms by his sides, transfer your hand to the back of his forearm immediately proximal to the wrist and ask him to straighten his arm while you try to bend it.

Wrists, fingers and thumbs

● For all the tests that follow on the arms, ask the patient to keep both elbows flexed to 90° with his arms by his sides and the forearms, wrists and hands extended in a straight line in front of him with the palms facing downwards in the prone position, unless otherwise stated.

● Test one joint at a time for both flexion and extension and any other movements, and then repeat the tests on the opposite arm.

For the *wrists*:

● **Flexors** (flexors carpi radialis and ulnaris): ask the patient to make both hands into tightly clenched fists. Now anchor one of his forearms by gripping it above the wrist with one of your hands, then ask him to bend his hand downwards while you try to extend it upwards by pushing upwards on its under side with your other hand.

● **Extensors** (extensors carpi radialis longus, brevis and ulnaris): while still anchoring the forearm by gripping it above the wrist, ask the patient to bend his hand backwards as far as he can while you try to flex it downwards by pushing down on the back of it with your other hand (Fig. 13.2).

For the *hands*:

● **Flexors** (flexors digitorum superficialis and profundus): ask the patient to oppose you while you try to open his fist. Then cross the index and middle index fingers of your uncommitted hand and ask the patient to grip them as hard as he can.

● **Extensors** (extensor digitorum): ask the patient to straighten his fingers, and then anchor his hand at the metacarpals by gripping them with one of your hands. Now ask him to keep his fingers straight while you try to flex them by bending them downwards with your other hand.

● **Abductors** (dorsal interosseus muscles): while the patient's fingers are still in the prone position and the wrists, hands and fingers are still in a straight line, ask him to spread (abduct) the fingers of one of his hands and try to oppose you as you squeeze them together.

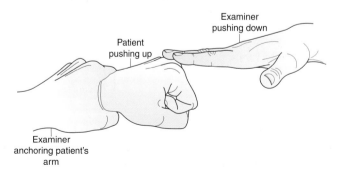

Fig 13.2 Testing the power of extension of the wrist

The letters in italic of the words *d*orsal and a*b*ductors go together to give the aid-to-memory '*DAB*'.

- **Adductors** (palmar interosseus muscles): now ask the patient to tightly grip a piece of paper between two of the fingers of one of his hands and keep the wrist, hand and fingers in a straight line while you try to pull it free.

The letters in italic of the words *p*almar and a*d*ductors go together to give the aid-to-memory '*PAD*'.

In summary, PAD = adductors and DAB = abductors.

For the *thumb*:

- Ask the patient to turn his hand over into the supine position with his fingers and hand facing upwards; then anchor his hand by gripping it at the wrist with your left hand and use your right hand for the following tests (Fig. 13.3).

- **Opposition**: ask the patient to keep his thumb straight and move it across his palm until the tip of it is against the base of the little finger of the same hand while you try to push it back.

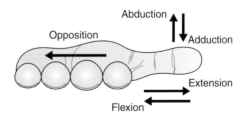

Fig 13.3 Movements of the thumb

- **Extension**: ask the patient to move his thumb out laterally in the plane of the palm while you try to oppose him.

- **Flexion**: ask the patient to straighten his thumb in the plane of the palm and then flex its distal joint (i.e. bend it) while you try to straighten it.

- **Abduction**: ask the patient to lift his thumb in a direction 90° away from the plane of the palm while you try to oppose him by pushing down on its upper side.

- **Adduction**: while the thumb is still abducted, ask the patient to return it to the plane of the palm while you try to oppose him by pulling up on its under side.

Muscles of the leg

- Ask the patient to either lie in the supine position or sit with his legs dangling over the end of the examination table.

Hips

Test both flexion and extension on one side, and then repeat both tests on the other side.

- **Flexion** (mainly iliopsoas): Ask the patient to bend one of his hips while you try to oppose him by pushing down on his lower thigh.

- **Hip extension** (gluteal muscles): Ask the patient to keep his hip on the table while you try to bend it by placing a hand behind his lower thigh and then lifting.

- **Abduction of the thigh** (gluteal muscles; test both sides simultaneously): Ask the patient to pull his legs apart while you oppose him by pushing in with a hand placed on the lateral side of each lower thigh.

- **Adduction of the thigh** (adductor magnus; test both sides simultaneously): Ask the patient to pull his legs together while you try to pull them apart with a hand placed on the medial side of each lower thigh.

Knee

Test both extension and flexion on one side, and then test both on the other side.

Extension (quadriceps muscles) and flexion (hamstring muscles):

- Ask the patient to flex one hip and knee but keep his foot on the examination table or, if he is sitting, to relax with his leg dangling.

- **Extension**: now place your right hand on the front of the lower part of his tibia and ask him to oppose you by trying to straighten his leg while you push and try to bend it more. If necessary, place your left hand on his knee to steady it.

- **Flexion**: while if necessary still steadying the knee with your left hand, move your right hand from the front to the back of the lower calf and ask the patient to oppose you and bend his leg more as you try to straighten it.

Feet

- For all these tests, ask the patient to continue sitting, or straighten his legs if he is lying supine. In either case, ask him to adjust the position of his feet so that they are at 90° to the lower part of his legs.

Dorsiflexion (mainly tibialis anterior, extensor hallucis longus and extensor digitorum longus); plantar flexion (mainly gastrocnemius and soleus):

- Test dorsiflexion/plantarflexion on one side, and then on the other. Then repeat the same sequence for eversion/inversion.

- **Dorsiflexion**: Place your fingers flat across the dorsum of one the patient's feet and ask him to bend his foot up while you try to push it down and plantarflex it.

- **Plantarflexion**: Now place your fingers flat across the distal part of the sole of one of the patient's feet and ask him to bend his foot down while you push up and try to dorsiflex it.

Eversion and inversion:

● **Eversion**: Anchor the patient's ankle with your left hand and place your right hand against the distal part of his foot on its lateral side. Ask the patient to twist his foot out and oppose you while you try to twist it medially with your right hand.

● **Inversion**: Repeat by placing your hand against the distal part of the foot on its medial side and ask the patient to twist his foot in and oppose you as you try to twist his foot laterally with your right hand.

Coordination: tests of the cerebellum

> **Note!**
>
> All these tests rely on an intact motor and sensory system. Signs of cerebellar disease are given in Box 13.2.

Box 13.2: Main signs of cerebellar disease

● Wide-based, unsteady gait
● Nystagmus – typically to the same side as the lesion
● Incoordination with an intention tremor on the same side as the lesion – best demonstrated by the finger/nose test
● Decreased muscle tone on the same side as the lesion
● Decreased reflexes on the same side as the lesion

Testing for nystagmus

● Stand about 1 m in front of the patient and ask him to keep his head still. Now place the index finger of your right hand about 30 cm in front of his eyes and ask him to follow it with his eyes as you move your finger, first to about 30 cm lateral to his right eye, then to about 30 cm lateral to his left eye, and finally back to the centre and upwards. At the extreme of each movement, stop for about 5 seconds, as any nystagmus that may be present may have a latent period or delay of onset of about 5 seconds.

Note!

Background information about nystagmus is on page 180.

Arms

● Ask the patient to perform each of these tests as quickly as possible on one arm then on the other.

Finger tapping

● Ask the patient to tap the back of one hand with the extended fingers of the other hand. Alternatively, so you can hear as well as see the response, you may ask the patient to tap a hollow object, such as a box, instead of the back of his hand.

Pronation/supination

● Ask the patient to alternately supinate/pronate one hand against the back of the other hand or against a hollow object such as a box.

'Piano playing'

● Ask the patient to place the tip of one of his thumbs against the tip of the index finger of the same hand. Now ask him to move the tip of the thumb from the tip of one finger to another of the same hand as quickly as possible, repeating several times.

Finger/nose test (test for intention tremor)

● Stand about 1.3 m in front of the patient and hold your right index finger up at the level of his face, about half way between the two of you. Now ask him to touch your finger with the index finger of one of his hands and take it back to his nose. Ask him to repeat the procedure several times as you move your finger from one position to another in front of him.

● Perform a similar test while the patient's eyes are shut. To do this, while the patient's eyes are still open and he is watching you, move your arm slightly to the side of his face and keep it in the same position. Now ask him to touch your index finger with his index finger. Then ask him to close his eyes and move his finger back to his nose. Now ask him to move his finger back and forwards and touch your finger and his nose several times while his eyes remain shut and your finger remains stationary.

● Overshooting or worsening of any tremor as the target is approached is known as an *intention tremor* and is suggestive of cerebellar disease.

Legs

● Ask the patient to either sit with his legs dangling or lie supine. Then repeat each of the following tests on one leg then on the other.

Heel/shin test

● Ask the patient to run the heel of one leg along the shin of the other leg as accurately as possible. Inability to perform this test accurately is suggestive of cerebellar disease, although allowance must be made for the age of the patient.

Toe-tapping test

● Place the palm of your right hand against the distal part of the sole of one of the patient's feet and ask him to tap your hand with his toes as fast as he can. Inability to perform this test accurately is suggestive of cerebellar disease.

Gait

Gait is usually assessed by performing three or four of the following tests.

Walking test

- Ask the patient to walk up and down the examination room and observe his bearing, arm swinging and gait. Examples of common abnormalities of gait are given on page 39.

- A broad-based, unsteady gait is suggestive of cerebellar disease. Slowness in starting and failure to swing the arms (i.e. bradykinesia and poverty of movement) is suggestive of Parkinson's disease (see page 40).

> **Note!**
>
> Several of the tests in this section, including this one, are commonly used to test for suspected drunkenness.

Heel/toe test (also known as tandem walking)

- Ask the patient to walk by placing the heel of one foot immediately in front of the toes of the other foot, and continue to walk in this fashion.

- Inability to perform this test accurately or a tendency to fall is suggestive of cerebellar disease.

Walking on toes test

- Ask the patient to walk as high up on his toes as possible.

- Inability to perform this test accurately or a tendency to fall is suggestive of cerebellar disease or weakness of the plantar flexor muscles of the foot.

Walking on heels test

- Ask the patient to walk on his heels.

- Inability to perform this test accurately or a tendency to fall is suggestive of cerebellar disease or weakness of the dorsiflexor muscles of the foot.

Hopping on one leg test

- Ask the patient to hop first on one leg and then on the other.

- Inability to perform this test accurately or a tendency to fall is compatible with cerebellar disease, although allowance must be made for the age of the patient.

Shallow knee-bend test

- Ask the patient to raise one foot off the ground and then do a shallow knee bend with the opposite leg.

- A tendency to fall is compatible with cerebellar disease or weakness of the proximal muscles of the leg, although allowance must be made for the age of the patient.

- Repeat on the opposite leg.

Romberg test

- Do this test first with the patient's eyes open and then with his eyes closed. With the eyes open, this is a test of coordination.

- Ask the patient to stand upright with his feet together and his arms by his sides.

- Failure to maintain this position for 20–30 seconds is suggestive of cerebellar disease.

- Repeat the test with the eyes closed.

- The test is now a test of position sense as well as coordination, as the patient is no longer able to use his vision to determine the position of his body.

Other tests of the limbs

Pronator drift test

- Ask the patient to stand with his eyes closed and his arms extended and pronated in front of him (i.e. palms facing downwards).

- The falling away of an arm (arm drift) suggests weakness or sensory loss of the limb due to hemiparesis or a musculoskeletal problem of the shoulder.

Tapping the extended arm test

● After performing the pronator drift test, and while the patient's eyes are still closed, gently tap the extended arm so that it is displaced downwards.

● Failure to reflexly return the arm to its previous position is compatible with weakness or sensory loss and is a common sign of hemiparesis.

● Repeat on the other arm.

Reflexes

Remember to ask the patient to relax, and remember that you must use a reflex hammer properly. Do not place your index finger along the shaft of the hammer handle. Instead, one of the best ways of eliciting the reflexes is to hold the end of the handle between the outer side of the index finger and the tip of the thumb of your dominant hand and swing the hammer with the wrist, letting the hammerhead perform most of the work (Fig. 13.4).

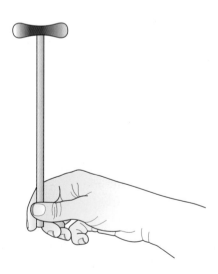

Fig 13.4 Holding a reflex hammer

Monitor the response by both *seeing* and *feeling* the resultant muscle contraction. Interpretation of the reflexes is discussed at the end of this chapter.

> If you wish to perfect the technique of doing reflexes, practise by holding the reflex hammer in your dominant hand as described above, and grip and anchor your wrist with your non-dominant hand, so that when you swing the hammer you are able to move only your wrist and the head of the hammer. Now pick a spot on a table and take a relaxed swing at it, letting your wrist and the head of the hammer do the work of striking the spot.

Arms

Perform each of the following tests on one side and then on the other.

Biceps (C5, C6)

- Ask the patient to rest his hands on his lap if he is sitting, or on his abdomen if he is lying supine.

- Then stretch the biceps tendon with the thumb or index finger of your non-dominant hand and strike your thumb or finger with the hammer.

Brachioradialis or radial (C7, C8)

- Hold the patient's arm flexed to about 90° in your non-dominant hand, or alternatively let his arm rest in a relaxed position on his lap or abdomen.

- Now strike the brachioradialis tendon on the lateral surface of the radius about 5–8 cm above the radial stylus.

Triceps (C6, C7, C8)

- You can perform this test in one of two ways. Either ask the patient to flex his elbow to about 90° and let you support his arm at the wrist with your non-dominant hand, or ask him to abduct his arm to shoulder level and let you grasp and bear the weight of his upper arm while his forearm hangs vertically free.

● Now strike the triceps tendon about 2–3 cm above the olecranon.

Legs

Perform each of the following tests on one leg and then on the other.

Quadruceps (L2, L3, L4)

● The patient should be either sitting with his legs dangling or, if lying flat, with his legs flexed and his feet on the examination table, with you supporting the weight of his legs by placing your non-dominant hand behind his knees. Now identify one of the patellar tendons as it lies between the patella and tibial tuberosity, and strike it with the head of the hammer.

Ankle (S1, S2)

● This test may be performed in any one of three positions. First, it can be done with the patient lying supine with his hip and knee flexed, his foot on the examination table and his knee flopping out laterally. Alternatively, it may be performed with the patient lying supine, the hip and knee flexed, the foot on the examination table and, for modesty, the knee *adducted* against the other leg. Finally, it may be tested with the patient sitting and the legs dangling.

● Having adopted a position, first gently dorsiflex the foot with your non-dominant hand to stretch the tendon, and then strike it with the head of the hammer at right angles to the line of the tendon.

Ankle clonus

● This is a sign of a hyperactive nervous system and can be performed in any of the three positions adopted for the ankle reflex.

- Ask the patient to relax, and then take hold of his foot and alternately dorsiflex and plantarflex it several times before sharply dorsiflexing it. If the patient has ankle clonus, the foot will continue to oscillate spontaneously between dorsiflexion and plantarflexion while you maintain it in dorsiflexion. One or two beats of clonus is normal, especially in people who are anxious; more prolonged clonus is suggestive of an UMN lesion.

Plantar reflex (Babinski response)

- Use the point of a key or the pointed end of the handle of a reflex hammer to *slowly* stroke the *outer side* of the sole of one of the patient's feet, starting near the heel and finishing by stroking across the ball of the foot.

- Normally, the toes either turn down or fail to respond. An upgoing response of the big toe, with or without fanning of the other toes, indicates an UMN lesion.

Abdominal reflexes

- With the patient relaxed in the supine position, stroke each quadrant of the abdomen with the pointed end of the handle of a reflex hammer and observe the resulting contraction of the abdominal muscles.

BACKGROUND INFORMATION

Reflexes

The reflexes are increased in UMN lesions and decreased in LMN and cerebellar lesions. The differences between an UMN lesion and a LMN lesion are listed in Box 13.3.

> **Box 13.3: Differences between an upper and a lower motor neurone lesion**
>
> | **Upper motor neurone** | **Lower motor neurone** |
> |---|---|
> | ● Weakness | Weakness |
> | ● Little or no wasting | Wasting + |
> | ● Increased tone (after a variable period of flaccidity) | Decreased tone (due to damage of the reflex arc) |
> | ● Increased reflexes (after being decreased at first) | Decreased reflexes (due to damage of the reflex arc) |
> | ● Extensor plantar reflex (positive Babinski) | Plantar reflex normal (i.e. flexor or absent) |
> | ● No fasciculation | Fasciculation + (due to denervation; page 190) |

The word 'brisk' is usually used to mean the size of a reflex rather than its speed. The speed is referred to by saying it is normal, slow or fast.

The ankle reflex, *and only the ankle reflex*, may be used (because it has the longest reflex arc in the body) to assess thyroid status. The ankle reflex is *fast* in hyperthyroidism and *slow* (particularly the relaxation phase) in hypothyroidism.

An individual reflex may be absent when the reflex arc supplying it is damaged. This occurs most commonly with sciatica and damage of the nerves S1 and S2 as they leave the spine, and results in an absent ankle reflex. The biceps, brachioradialis and triceps reflexes may also be absent if their respective nerves and reflex arcs are damaged by pathology in the neck, most commonly as a result of trauma or degenerative disease due to advancing age affecting the bones and intervertebral discs in the neck.

Reinforcement of the reflexes

If the reflexes are reduced or difficult to demonstrate, ask the patient to clench his teeth while you try to elicit the arm reflexes; in the case of the leg reflexes, ask the patient to curve the fingers of one hand around the fingers of the other hand and pull on them while you try to elicit the reflexes.

Finally, Box 13.4 describes the differences between a peripheral neuropathy and a typical myopathy

---

Box 13.4 Clinical differences between a peripheral neuropathy and a typical myopathy

Peripheral neuropathy	Myopathy
● Typically peripheral	Typically proximal
● Muscle wasting +	Muscle bulk typically relatively preserved
● Reflexes decreased or absent	Reflexes decreased but relatively preserved
● Fasciculation + (page 190)	No fasciculation
● Sensory loss often present	No sensory loss

14

SENSORY SYSTEM

Equipment needed

- Two pins or safety-pins or a paperclip
- Piece of cotton wool or a Q-tip
- Turning fork (the best tuning forks vibrate at 128 or 256Hz)
- Test tubes containing cold and warm water
- Familiar objects such as coins, a pen, a watch and a key

Note!

Before each test, carefully explain to the patient what you are about to do, and that when it involves using a pin, you will not hurt him.

Position of the patient

- The patient should be either sitting or lying supine in warm, quiet surroundings

Order of the examination and list of parameters to be tested

- Light touch and pinprick sense

- Position sense
- Vibration sense
- Temperature sense
- Stereognosis (the ability to recognize objects by touch)
- Object recognition
  - ○ Number recognition
  - ○ Two-point discrimination
  - ○ Point localization
  - ○ Extinction

EXAMINATION

Light touch and pinprick

- Use the point of a pin or safety-pin applied lightly at 90° to the patient's skin to test pinprick, and a piece of cotton wool or a Q-tip to test light touch.

- The best technique is to touch each site two or three times in quick succession, so that the patient has a good chance to recognize the stimulus.

- Ask the patient to close his eyes or look up at the ceiling and place his hands in the supine position with the fingers extended.

- Start distally and randomly touch the distal pads of the thumb and one or two fingers of one hand with either the pin or the cotton. After each stimulus, ask the patient which he feels. Then repeat the tests on the other hand.

- Now, comparing one side with the other, test two or three sites further up each arm.

- Repeat on the big toes, the dorsums of both feet and further up the legs, comparing one side with the other, and finally test one or two areas on the trunk.

> ## Note!
>
> Never use a blood-taking or injection needle for sensory testing, as they are very sharp and draw blood – and the patient won't be very pleased with you!

Position sense

● Ask the patient to turn his hands into the prone position. Then gently grip the *sides* of one of the patient's thumbs between your index finger and thumb, and ask the patient to close his eyes or look up at the ceiling.

● Now move the thumb up or down a little to a new position. Ask the patient which way it moved.

● Check the result by moving the thumb in the opposite direction.

● Repeat the test on the opposite thumb and on one or two fingers on each side, and then bilaterally on the big toes.

● Patients are normally very sensitive and are able to detect movements of just a few millimetres.

● If the patient cannot detect movement in the periphery, work proximally, testing movements of the wrists and. if necessary, the elbows, ankles and knees.

Vibration sense

● When performing this test, ask the patient what he feels, as that is an open question, rather than whether the tuning fork is vibrating, which is a closed question.

● Ask the patient to close his eyes or look up at the ceiling.

● Set the fork vibrating by striking it on a solid object such a table.

● Place the vibrating fork on the distal pad or a bony prominence on one of the patient's fingers and ask him what he feels. Repeat on the adjacent thumb and then on the thumb and a finger of the opposite hand.

- If the patient does not feel the vibration, move proximally to the bony prominences of, first, the wrists and, if necessary, the elbows.

- Repeat the test on the big toes of both feet. If the patient does not feel a vibration in the toes, move proximally to the ankles and, if necessary, the upper tibia. Bear in mind, however, that vibration sense tends to decrease with age.

- At one or two sites, test the accuracy of the patient's response by stopping (i.e. extinguishing) the vibration surreptitiously. Do this by gripping the vibrating arms of the fork with your fingers and asking the patient what he feels. Without seeing or knowing what you have done, the patient should be able to tell you that he no longer feels the vibration. If necessary, ask him whether or not the fork is still vibrating.

Temperature sense

- Ask the patient to close his eyes or look up at the ceiling and tell you whether he feels something hot or cold as you randomly lay the side of a test tube containing either cold or warm water first on one forearm, then on the other, and then on one shin and then the other. If test tubes of water are not available, test for cold by using the side of a tuning fork or the metal handle of a reflex hammer.

Stereognosis

- This is the ability to recognize objects by touch, and is tested on one side and then the other.

- These tests require the ability to integrate information and are therefore tests of parietal function. They also require an intact peripheral sensory system.

Object recognition

● Tell the patient that you are about to place a common object in his hand and that he may use his fingers to identify it. Then ask him to close his eyes or look up at the ceiling. Now place a common object such as a coin, a pen, a key, a paperclip or a watch in his palm. Ask him what it is. Then repeat with other objects on the list.

Number recognition

● Ask the patient to close his eyes or look up at the ceiling, and place his hands in the supine position with the palms open.

● Now ask him to tell you which number from 0 to 9 you are writing as you write on one of his palms with either the retracted point of a ballpoint pen, the point of a key or the pointed end of the handle of a reflex hammer. Alternatively, write on the front of his forearms.

Two-point discrimination

● Ask the patient to close his eyes or look up at the ceiling, and place his hands in the supine position with the fingers extended.

● Now ask him to tell you how many pins or points he feels as you randomly and lightly touch the distal pad of one of his fingers with either one or two pins, or one or both points of an opened paperclip.

● Start with a distance of about 1 cm between the two pins or points, and gradually reduce the distance until the patient can no longer discriminate between them.

● Patients can usually differentiate between one and two points placed as close as 2–3 mm apart on the pads of the fingers or the thumb.

● Repeat on the distal pad of another finger, and then on the thumb and one or two fingers of the opposite hand.

● Now test the dorsums of the feet.

- Patients usually require 5 mm or more to discriminate between two points on the feet (or other parts of the body) as innervation to the foot and other areas is not as rich as to the fingers.

Point localization

- Ask the patient to close his eyes and point to each place you touch with your finger as you touch various points on his arms, legs and trunk.

Extinction

- Ask the patient to close his eyes and place his arms in the supine position with the fingers extended. Then ask him to tell you which of his arms you have touched as you touch first one of his forearms and then the other.
- Then touch both forearms simultaneously.
- Patients are normally able to recognize both the individual and the combined stimuli. Assuming that the patient has an intact peripheral sensory system, those who miss the stimulus on one side when both arms are touched simultaneously usually have partial loss of function of the parietal lobe on the opposite side.

Special sensory tests for meningeal irritation

- **Brazinski sign:** with the patient in the supine position, gently flex his neck. The test is positive if the patient flexes his hips and knees.
- **Kernig's sign:** with the patient in the supine position, gently lift his legs straight up. The test is positive if the patient complains of pain in the neck.

BACKGROUND INFORMATION

Sensory testing

Light touch, position and vibration senses are conducted up in the dorsal columns and cross over to the opposite side in the brainstem.

From the neck upwards, the *central* part of the dorsal columns contains fibres from the legs and lower part of the trunk in a tract known as in the *fasciculus gracilis*, whereas the *outer* part of the column contains fibres from the arms and upper part of the trunk that run up in a tract known as the *fasciculus cuneatus* (Fig. 14.1).

Pain, temperature and coarse touch sensation cross over almost immediately after entering the spinal cord and are conducted up in the *lateral spinothalamic tracts* of the opposite side.

Loss of light touch, position and vibration sensation occur with peripheral neuropathy and disease of the dorsal columns. Loss of pain and temperature sensation occur with peripheral neuropathy and disease of the lateral spinothalamic tracts.

Simplified way of remembering the dermatomes on the front of the body and perineum

Reference dermatomes

● The method described here for remembering the dermatomes relies on committing a small number of reference dermatomes to memory, as listed below and illustrated in Fig. 14.2
  ○ C4 = the dermatome innervating the lower part of the neck immediately above the clavicles, including the skin over the front of the trapezius muscles.

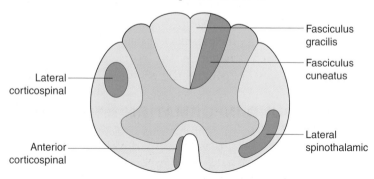

Fig 14.1 Motor and sensory tracts in the spinal cord

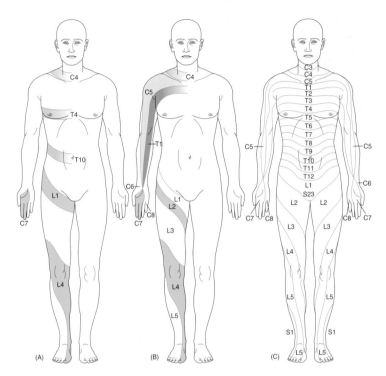

Fig 14.2 (A) Reference dermatomes. (B) Dermatomes of the arms and legs. (C) Dermatomes on the front of the body

○ C7 = the dermatome innervating the index and middle fingers. This is most easily remembered by the fact that when extended on their own, these two fingers look like the barrel of a revolver.

○ T4 = the dermatome across the chest at the level of the nipple.

○ T10 = the dermatome across the abdomen at the level of the umbilicus.

○ L1 = the dermatome sloping down along the groin.

○ L4 = the dermatome sloping down across the knee.

○ S1 and S2 = the dermatomes innervating the sole of the foot and back of the leg.

Note of caution!

Beneath the reference dermatome C4, which innervates the lower part of the neck, is C5, the lowest cervical dermatome to be represented on the front of the chest. Immediately beneath C5 are T1, T2 and T3, followed by T4, the reference dermatome across the chest at the level of the nipple.

The dermatomes missing from the front of the chest, that is, C6–C8, are represented on the back, the backs of the arms and on the fingers, where they include the reference dermatome C7, mentioned on page 221.

Tip about the dermatomes of the leg

The easiest way to remember the direction of L1 is to run your hand down along your own groin; and for L4, to run your hand obliquely down across your knee from the lateral side of the lower thigh to the medial side of the lower leg.

By using the reference dermatomes described on page 220 and by referring to the accompanying diagrams, it is a relatively easy matter to insert the remaining dermatomes as follows.

Hand

By using C7 as the reference dermatome from which to count in either direction, the innervation of the thumb is C6, and that of the fourth and fifth fingers is C8, (see Fig. 14.2B).

Anterolateral aspect of the arm

Counting back from the reference dermatome C7 (the index and middle fingers), the innervation of the thumb is C6, as stated immediately above, and of that of the antero-lateral aspect of the arm is the next nerve up to emerge from the spinal cord, namely C5, (see Fig. 14.2B).

Anteromedial aspect of the arm

Counting from the reference dermatome C7, the innervation of the fourth and fifth fingers is C8, and of that of the *anteromedial aspect of the arm* is the next nerve down to emerge from the spinal chord, namely T1, (see Fig. 14.2B).

Front of the chest above the nipple

The dermatome supplying the upper part of the *neck* above the reference dermatome C4 is C3. On the uppermost part of the chest, the dermatomes C6, C7 and C8 are missing, as explained in the paragraph on the previous page entitled *Note of caution*. The dermatomes between the reference dermatomes C4 above the clavicle and T4 at the level of the nipple are therefore C5, T1, T2 and T3, (see Fig. 14.2C).

Front of the chest and abdomen from the nipple to the groin

T5–T9 are easily inserted between the reference dermatome T4 at the nipple and the reference dermatome T10 at the umbilicus. In the lower abdomen, it is also an easy matter to insert dermatomes T11 and T12 between the reference dermatome T10 at the umbilicus and the reference dermatome L1 in the groin, (see Fig. 14.2C).

Leg

Thigh

The dermatomes in the middle of the thigh, between the reference dermatomes L1 in the groin and L4 at the knee, are L2 and L3, (see Fig. 14.2B).

Lower leg and upper surface the foot

As you slide your hand down across your knee over the reference dermatome L4, it ends up on the medial side of the lower leg, which it supplies together with the upper medial surface of the foot. Lateral to L4 is L5, supplying the lateral side of the lower leg and the upper lateral surface of the foot, (see Fig. 14.2B).

Sole of the foot and back of the leg

As stated on page 221 in the paragraph entitled 'Reference dermatomes', the dermatomes supplying the sole of the foot and back of the leg are the reference dermatomes S1and S2.

Perineum

From the back of the leg, the reference dermatomes S1and S2 form *a semicircle round the periphery of the perineum* and then descend down the opposite leg to the sole of the foot. Inside the semicircle formed by S1and S2, S3–S5 form concentric circles around the anus, with S2 and S3 supplying the genitalia at the front, (see Fig. 14.2C).

Using knowledge of the dermatomes in clinical practice

The level of a lesion in the spinal cord may be established clinically by advising the patient about what you intend to do and then asking him to tell you when he feels a change of sensation as you do the following. Gently run the point of a pin or a safety pin first down one side of the front of his trunk and then down the other. The level at which the patient reports sensation has changed corresponds to the dermatome at the level of the lesion. Similarly, the dermatome involved in sensory loss in a limb may be established by gently exploring pain sensation with the point of a pin or a safety pin.

15

UNCONSCIOUS
PATIENT

BACKGROUND INFORMATION

As full a history as possible should be obtained from anyone who saw the patient at the beginning of the episode or anyone who knows him. In particular, information should be sought about the cause and duration of the unconsciousness, including enquiring into such factors as drugs, alcohol, trauma, epilepsy, preceding chest pain or headache, and whether the patient has ever suffered unconsciousness before (Box 15.1).

EXAMINATION

Full examination of every system of the body is required, in particular assessing:

- **The patient's posture**
  - **Decorticate:** this is a posture in which the patient lies with the arms flexed and adducted and the legs extended; it is usually due to a large cerebral vascular accident affecting the cerebral white matter, internal capsule or thalamus.
  - **Decerebrate:** this is a posture in which the patient is in opisthotonos with his back arched by spasm and his

Box 15.1: Causes of unconsciousness

Structural brain causes
- Large cerebral hemisphere lesion, e.g. stroke, tumour, abscess
- Bilateral cerebral disease, e.g. encephalitis
- Head injury
- Extradural haemorrhage
- Subdural haemorrhage
- Subarachnoid haemorrhage
- Brainstem lesion, e.g. stroke

Other neurological causes
- Epilepsy (Box 15.2)

Metabolic
- Hypoglycaemia
- Hyperglycaemia
- Severe uraemia
- Hypothermia
- Hypothyroidism
- Hepatic encephalopathy
- Metabolic acidosis
- Severe carbon dioxide retention
- Hyponatraemia
- Drugs
  - Therapeutic: anaesthetics, sedatives, hypoglycaemics, antidepressants
  - Drug abuse: opiates, alcohol

Cardiac causes
Asystole, ventricular fibrillation
Ventricular tachycardia
Aortic stenosis
Vasovagal attack
Orthostatic hypotension

Other causes
Psychological

jaws clenched, his arms extended, adducted and internally rotated, and his legs and feet extended. It is usually due to a midbrain or brainstem lesion.

- **Level of consciousness:** assess this using the Glasgow Coma Scale (Box 15.3, page 228).

- **Evidence of trauma:** look for bruising, bogginess of the scalp or misalignment of bones.

Box 15.2: Clinical features of a generalized tonic-clonic (grand mal) seizure

Aura (warning)
- A feeling in the epigastrium lasting a few seconds or minutes, or a partial seizure, such as a Jacksonian or temporal lobe seizure, progressing to a tonic-clonic seizure

Tonic phase
- This involves the brain stem and lasts for 30–60 seconds, and results in the patient becoming unconscious, falling to the ground and becoming rigid, spastic and cyanosed

Clonic phase
- In this phase, the patient jerks, often rhythmically for about 1–2 minutes
- He may also bite the lateral side of his tongue or be incontinent of urine

Coma
- This lasts from a few seconds to hours, during which the corneal reflex is absent and the plantar reflex is extensor

Post-ictal phase
- This is associated with sleep, headache and/or automatic behaviour

- **Odours:** note any odours such as the odour of alcohol, ketones or foetor hepaticus (the unpleasant odour of liver failure).

- **Body temperature:** check for hyperpyrexia and hypothermia.

- **Respiratory rate and pattern:** check the rate and regularity of the breathing, and note any Kussmaul acidotic breathing or Cheyne–Stokes respiration (see page 129).

- **Pulse and blood pressure:** Check to see if the pulse and blood pressure are recordable, or whether the blood pressure is abnormally high as occurs with some strokes and hypertensive encephalopathy.

- **Neck stiffness:** check for any stiffness suggesting meningitis or subarachnoid haemorrhage.

- **Pupil size and reaction to light:** check the pupils for size and regularity, and for whether they contract when a bright torch-light is shone into them. The following important reactions occur:
  - **Bilaterally normal pupils** reactive to light occur with metabolic coma.
  - **Bilaterally fixed dilated pupils** unresponsive to light occur with brainstem death.
  - **Bilaterally dilated pupils** slightly responsive to light occur with tricyclic antidepressant poisoning.
  - **Bilaterally fixed pinpoint pupils** occur with opiate poisoning and pontine stroke.
  - **Fixed dilatation of *one* pupil** occurs when the nucleus of cranial nerve III on one side is pushed against the tentorium by an extradural or subdural haemorrhage following trauma; it is an indication for emergency investigation and possible surgery.

- **Fundi:** check for papilloedema suggestive of raised intracranial pressure, or haemorrhages (known as subhyaloid haemorrhages) indicating that blood has tracked down to the eye in the cerebrospinal fluid as a result of a subarachnoid haemorrhage.

- **Movements of the eyes and limbs:** note any movement, and if so, whether it is unilateral or bilateral.

- **Limb reflexes:** test the limb reflexes and note whether they are present, and if so, whether they are equal on both sides and whether the plantar reflex is flexor or extensor.

Glasgow Coma Scale

- The Glasgow Coma Scale allows the depth and progress of the patient's condition to be monitored, and is particularly useful in cases of trauma to the head. Scores are listed in

Box 15.3. The scores for the three individual parts are added together. The minimum score is 3 and the maximum is 15.

Box 15.3: The Glasgow Coma Scale

	Patient's response	**Score**
Eye opening	Spontaneous	4
	To verbal command	3
	To pain	2
	No response	1
Verbal response	Orientated	5
	Confused speech	4
	Inappropriate speech	3
	Incomprehensible sounds	2
	No response	1
Motor response	Obeys	6
	Localizes	5
	Withdraws	4
	Flexion	3
	Extension	2
	No response	1

BRAINSTEM DEATH

Background information

The problem of deciding whether or not a patient is dead arises with those deeply unconscious patients who are on a mechanical ventilator and in whom, as a consequence, it is not known whether spontaneous breathing is possible, as that is one of the criteria of brainstem death.

In this situation, it has been found that the way to determine whether or not the patient is alive or dead is to test brainstem function via its reflexes.

First, however, the history, examination and investigations must all be carefully reviewed to exclude causes of unconsciousness that are reversible or treatable, such as surgically treatable head injury or intracranial haemorrhage, drug overdose and the metabolic conditions listed in Box 15.1 (page 226).

Examination

Assuming that treatable causes have been excluded, the following tests should be carried out and the results verified before brainstem death may be certified:

● The **pupillary reflex** must be absent to bright torch-light.

● The **corneal reflex** must be absent.

● The **vestibular–ocular reflex** must be absent, that is, there must be no movement of the eyes on instillation by syringe of 50 ml of ice-cold water into the external auditory meatus of each ear, after first checking that the meatus is clear of wax and foreign bodies.

● The **oculocephalic reflex** must be absent, that is, there must be no movement of the eyes when the head is rotated from side to side. In a comatose patient with an intact brainstem, the eyes rotate and remain pointing in the original direction (doll's eye movement); with brainstem death, the eyes do not move.

● **Cranial nerves**: there must be no contraction of the facial muscles when a painful stimulus is applied to the forehead.

● **Gag reflex**: there must be no response when the back of the pharynx and the trachea are stimulated with a suction tube.

● **Respiratory response to hypercapnoea**: there must be no response when the ventilator is disconnected for up to 10 minutes after first administering 5 per cent carbon dioxide and 95 per cent oxygen via the ventilator for 5 minutes. During the period that the ventilator is disconnected, the patient should receive 100 per cent oxygen via a tracheal catheter inserted into the endotracheal tube, and should have blood gases measured to establish that the arterial partial pressure of carbon dioxide has risen sufficiently high (>6.7 kPa) to stimulate any possible ventilation.

16

MUSCULOSKELETAL SYSTEM

Equipment needed

● Tape measure

Notes about examination of the musculoskeletal system

● The musculoskeletal system is concerned mainly with joints, bones, tendons and ligaments. Muscle power is examined as part the central nervous system.
● Remember to examine both sides of the body.

Position of the patient

● The patient should be sitting or standing in warm quiet surroundings

Order of the examination

● Inspection
● Palpation
● Range of motion.

> **Note!**
>
> When testing range of motion, it may help if you demonstrate each movement you want the patient to make by doing it yourself as you ask him to do it.

BACKGROUND INFORMATION

Inspection

When examining the musculoskeletal system look for *redness, swelling, muscular wasting or deformity of the limbs.*

> **Note!**
>
> - **Redness** of the skin overlying a joint may be due to inflammation or arthritis.
> - **Swelling** in or around a joint may be due to infection, trauma, thickening of the synovial membrane, effusion or bony hypertrophy.
> - **Deformity** may be due to fracture of a bone, muscle spasm, dislocation of a joint, which is defined as a *complete* loss of contact between the two surfaces of a joint, or subluxation, which is defined as a *partial* loss of contact (Fig. 16.1). *Symmetrical deformity* of the hands with swelling, subluxation and ulnar deviation is typical of rheumatoid arthritis.

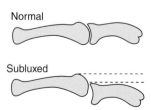

Fig 16.1 Subluxation

Palpation

When palpating, palpate with your thumbs and fingers and note any *tenderness, swelling, unusual warmth or crepitus.*

> **Note!**
>
> - **Tenderness and pain** may be due to pathology in a joint, trauma, tendonitis, bursitis or osteomyelitis (Box 16.1).
> - **Swelling**: this is discussed on the previous page in the notes about inspection.
> - **Unusual warmth**: this suggests inflammation.
> - **Crepitus**: this is a palpable or audible crunching due to the worn, roughened surfaces of a joint rubbing together as it moves. Crepitus occurs in conditions such as osteoarthritis and rheumatoid arthritis, and also occasionally with fractures.

> **Box 16.1: Causes of pain and tenderness in a joint**
>
> - **Inflammation of the synovium**, e.g. rheumatoid arthritis or systemic lupus erythematosus
> - **Mechanical causes**, e.g. trauma or osteoarthritis
> - **Infection** due to pyogenic bacteria, such as *Staphylococcus aureus*, *Salmonella typhi*, *Neisseria gonorrhoeae* or non-pyogenic bacteria, e.g. *Mycobacterium tuberculosis*

Range of motion

When testing the range of motion, note any instability, reduction or increase in the range of motion of a joint. Decreased range occurs with arthritis, inflammation and bony fixation.

EXAMINATION

Temporomandibular joint

- For inspection and palpation, position yourself in front of the patient.

Inspection

● Inspect both joints for any redness, swelling or deformity.

Palpation

● Palpate both joints at the same time with the tips of your index fingers, feeling for any swelling or tenderness.

● Ask the patient to open and close his mouth. Your fingers should fall into the joint space as the mouth opens. Check whether the range of motion is smooth. Clicking as the joint moves is normal.

Range of motion

Ask the patient to demonstrate the following *three* movements:

● **Opening and closing**: the gap between the upper and lower teeth is normally between 3 and 6 cm when the mouth is fully open.

● **Protrusion and retraction**: the lower teeth can normally be protruded in front of the upper teeth.

● **Side-to-side motion**: this is usually 1–2 cm.

Arms

Shoulder

> **Warning**
>
> Examination of this joint is complex.

Inspection

This is performed on one shoulder and then the other.

Inspect the shoulder joint and shoulder muscles from both the front and the back, looking for the following:

● **Swelling** of the joint and subacromial bursa. The latter lies immediately beneath the acromion, which is a bony protrusion from the upper part of the scapula, lying above the shoulder at the lateral end of the clavicle, as illustrated in Fig. 16.2.

● **Muscle wasting**: if present, this is suggestive of denervation, cachexia or myopathy due, for instance, to hyperthyroidism.

● **Bony landmarks** (Fig. 16.2): look for swelling or deformity of the following:
  ○ **Clavicle**, to be found running medially from the front of the shoulder.
  ○ **Acromion**, which, as stated above, is a bony protrusion from the upper part of the scapula at the lateral end of the clavicle.
  ○ **Coracoid process**, which is a bony forward-pointing protrusion from the scapula, just medial to the head of the humerus and immediately beneath the lateral end of the clavicle. The coracoid process is attached by ligaments to the acromion, clavicle and shoulder

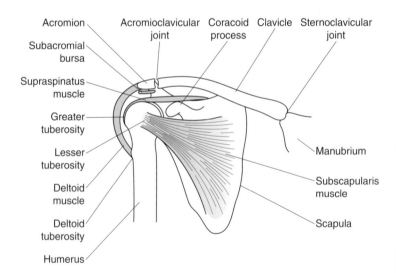

Fig 16.2 Bones of the shoulder from the front (adapted with kind permission from Abrahams P, Craven J and Lumley J, *Illustrated Clinical Anatomy*, Great Britain: Hodder Education, 2005).

capsule. The short head of biceps and the coracobrachialis muscles are also attached to it.

○ **Greater tubercle or tuberosity**, which is the point of insertion of three of the muscles of the rotator cuff, located on the *upper lateral* aspect of the humerus. (The rotator cuff is discussed below.)

Palpation

This is performed on one shoulder and then the other.

Identify and note any tenderness or swelling of the following:

● **Sternoclavicular joint** at the medial end of the clavicle.

● **Acromion** at the lateral end of the clavicle.

● **Subacromial bursa**: to bring the bursa into a position where it can be easily palpated, ask the patient to extend his arm backwards. This exposes the bursa beneath the front of the acromion. However, it is only palpable if it is inflamed.

● **Acromioclavicular joint**: use the tips of either your index or middle fingers to find and explore the joint, which lies between the lateral end of the clavicle and the medial end of the acromion.

● **Coracoid process**: ask the patient to extend his arm backwards to bring the coracoid process into a position where it can be easily palpated beneath the lateral end of the clavicle immediately medial to the head of the humerus.

> Both the subacromial bursa and the coracoid process are surprisingly high up relative to the head of the humerus.

● **Rotator cuff**: This consists of four muscles, three of which are inserted onto the greater tuberosity, which, as stated above and shown in Fig. 16.3, is located on the upper lateral side of the humerus. The easiest way to palpate the muscles is from behind the patient with his arm at his side. From this position, the three muscles inserted into the greater tuberosity from the top, going backwards and

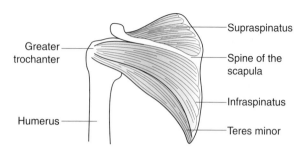

Fig 16.3 Back of the shoulder showing the rotator cuff

downwards are *supraspinatus*, which is inserted beneath the acromion, *infraspinatus*, which is inserted posteriorly to supraspinatus, and *teres minor*, which is inserted posteriorly and inferiorly to infraspinatus. A fourth muscle, *subscapularis*, passes both laterally and forwards from the anterior surface of the scapula to be inserted onto the lesser tuberosity on the front of the humerus. Pain and tenderness in the rotator cuff causes inability to raise the arm laterally to the level of the shoulder and occurs with tears, sprains or rupture of the tendons, most commonly of supraspinatus.

● **Biceps tendon:** Ask the patient to flex his elbow to 90° and rotate his arm laterally. The biceps tendon can now be palpated lying in the biceps groove on the anterior aspect of the upper humerus.

Range of motion

The patient should be standing for this.

Ask the patient to perform the following six movements on both arms simultaneously, as illustrated in Fig. 16.4:

● **Forward flexion:** start with his arms hanging down by the sides, and keeping them straight, raise them *forwards* until they are vertically over his head. (Normally, the range is 180°.)

● **Extension:** start with his arms hanging down by his sides and, keeping them straight, extend them backwards as far as they will go. (Normally the range is 50°.)

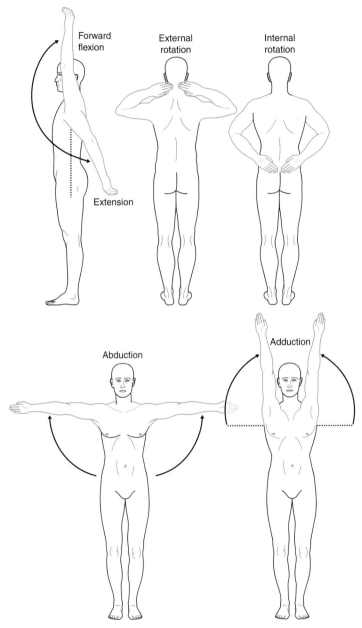

Fig 16.4 Range of motion of the shoulder

- **Abduction**: start with his arms hanging down by his sides, and, keeping them straight, raise them laterally to shoulder level with his palms facing down. This is a test of glenohumeral motion and is normally 90°.

- **Adduction**: start with his arms in the horizontal abducted position, and keeping them straight, raise them until they are vertically over his head, with his palms facing inwards. This is a test of both glenohumeral and scapulothoracic movement, and is called *adduction* because the movement is towards the midline. Normally, the range is 90°.

- **External rotation and abduction**: place both hands behind his neck with his elbows pointing sideway. (Normally the range is 90°.)

- **Internal rotation and adduction**: place both hands behind the small of his back. Normally, the range is 90°.

- An inability to perform these movements suggests muscle weakness, arthritis or inflammation of the joints, tendons or bursae.

Special tests for suspected damage of the rotator cuff

- Ask the patient to bend his elbow to 90° and keep his arm by his side with his forearm pointing forwards and his hand in the neutral vertical position midway between supination/pronation for each of these tests, which are demonstrated in Fig. 16.5. Pain occurring during a test indicates damage.

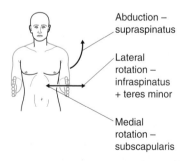

Abduction – supraspinatus

Lateral rotation – infraspinatus + teres minor

Medial rotation – subscapularis

Fig 16.5 Testing the muscles of the rotator cuff

- **Supraspinatus:** place a hand on the lateral side of the patient's elbow and ask him to lift his arm out (abduction) while you try to push it in.

- **Subscapularis:** place your hand against the medial side of the patient's wrist and ask him to rotate his arm medially while you try to rotate it laterally.

- **Infraspinatus and teres minor:** move your hand to the lateral side of the patient's wrist and ask him to rotate his arm out laterally while you try to push it medially.

Box 16.2: Common causes of a painful shoulder

Trauma
- Dislocation or fracture

Rotator cuff syndrome
- Tears, rupture or sprains associated with pain and tenderness over the insertion of the muscles of the rotator cuff with pain and limitation of movement on performing the special tests listed in the text

Acromioclavicular joint disease
- Osteoarthritis or inflammation of the ligaments stabilizing the joint

Glenohumeral disorders
- Osteoarthritis, or frozen shoulder, which is a condition associated with fibrosis and contraction of the anterior surface of the joint capsule that results in pain that is often worse at night, together with tenderness and slowly progressive stiffness of the shoulder and limited range of both passive and active movements, particularly external rotation

Referred pain from the neck
- Pain in the shoulder that is often associated with painful movements of the neck, pain radiating to the scapula and occasionally paraesthesiae in the arm

Referred pain from the diaphragm
- Pain in the shoulder that is due to conditions in the abdomen such as biliary colic and peritonitis

Elbows

Inspection

This is performed on one elbow after the other.

- Support the patient's forearm semi-flexed to about 70°.

- Identify and inspect the medial and lateral condyles of the humerus and the olecranon process of the ulnar at the back of the joint. Note any swelling or nodules, such as rheumatoid nodules or gouty tophi consisting of deposits of sodium urate crystals.

- Swelling and redness over the olecranon process occurs with *olecranon bursitis*.

Palpation

This is performed on one elbow after the other.

- Grasp the patient's wrist with your left hand and palpate the grooves between the epicondyles and the olecranon with your right hand, noting any tenderness, swelling or thickening.

- Tenderness over the lateral epicondyle is known as *tennis elbow*. Tenderness over the medial epicondyle is known as *golfer's elbow*.

Range of motion

This is performed on both sides simultaneously. Ask the patient to perform the following:

- **Flexion and extension**: bend and straighten the elbows as far as possible. Normally, the ranges are 160° and 180°, respectively.

- **Supination and pronation**: place the arms at the sides with the elbows flexed to 90° to minimize any shoulder movement; then turn the palms upwards (supination) and downwards (pronation). From the neutral midway position with the hands vertical, the range of each movement is normally 90°.

Wrists, hands, fingers and thumbs

Inspection

This is performed on one side and then on the other.

● Watch the way the patient moves his hands. Guarded movements suggest injury or arthritis.

● Inspect the palmar and dorsal surfaces of the wrists and fingers for redness, swelling or subluxation due to arthritis or misalignment suggestive of injury.

● Observe the thenar and hypothenar eminences and the spaces between the metacarpal bones for muscle wasting suggestive of a lesion of either the median or ulnar nerves.

Palpation

● Ask the patient to flex both his elbows to 90° with his arms by his side, his forearms straight out in front of him and his hands in the prone position. Perform all of the following tests first on one side and then on the other.

● **Palpation of the distal ends of the radius and ulna**: with your thumbs on top and your fingers underneath the wrist, palpate the distal ends of both the radius and the ulna. Tenderness or a 'step' in the distal end of the radius occurs with *Colles fracture.*

● **Palpation of the groove between the ends of the long bones and the wrist**: using the same technique as above, palpate for tenderness, unusual warmth, swelling or bogginess. Injury is usually unilateral; rheumatoid arthritis of the wrist is typically bilateral.

● **Palpation of the eight carpal bones**: these are immediately distal to the wrist. Compress each bone between your thumb and index fingers as you did for the ends of the long bones.

● **Palpation of the anatomical snuffbox**: find the anatomical snuffbox by asking the patient to extend his thumb, that is, move the thumb laterally in the plane of the palm. The snuffbox lies between the two tendons that become prominent at the base of the thumb. Tenderness in the anatomical snuffbox suggests a fracture of the scaphoid bone.

● **Palpation of the five metacarpal bones and the proximal, middle and distal phalanges of each finger:** gently compress each bone between your thumbs and index fingers, checking the metacarpophalangeal and interphalangeal joints of each finger and thumb for swelling, bogginess or tenderness suggestive of injury or arthritis. Note any *spindling* or *swan-neck* deformity due to rheumatoid arthritis (Box 16.2, see page 43). or Heberden's nodes due to osteoarthritis (see page 42).

Range of motion

This is performed on both sides simultaneously while the elbows are still flexed to 90° and the hands are initially in the prone position.

For the *wrists*:

● **Flexion:** ask the patient to flex his wrists downwards as far as possible. Normally this is 90°.

● **Extension:** ask the patient to extend his wrists backwards as far as possible. Normally this is 70°.

● **Ulnar and radial deviation:** ask the patient to move his wrists laterally and then medially as far as possible. Normally this is 55° to the ulnar side and 20° to the radial side.

For the *fingers*:

● **Flexion and extension:** ask the patient to make a tight fist with his thumbs across his knuckles.

● Now ask him to extend and spread his fingers. The fingers should open and close smoothly.

- Test extension and flexion of individual interphalangeal joints.

- **Abduction and adduction:** ask the patient to spread his fingers apart (abduction) and bring them together (adduction). Check that the movements are smooth and coordinated.

For the *thumbs* (see Fig, 13.3 on page 200):

- Now ask the patient to turn his hands into the *supine* position with the forearms, wrists and fingers extended in a straight line in front of him.

- **Flexion:** ask the patient to flex both joints of his thumbs.

- **Extension:** ask the patient to move his thumbs laterally as far as they will go in the plane of his palms.

- **Abduction and adduction:** ask the patient to move his thumbs as far as they will go at right angles from the plane of his palms, initially upwards (abduction) and then downwards (adduction).

- **Opposition:** ask the patient to keep his thumbs straight and place the tip of each of them against the base of his little fingers.

Tests for the carpal tunnel syndrome

This is performed on both wrists.

- **Phalen's test:** this is performed with the elbow flexed to about 90° and the hand in the prone position.

- Explain to the patient what you intend to do, and then flex and hold one of his wrists in acute flexion. Alternatively, ask the patient to flex both wrists simultaneously to a right angle and press the backs of both hands together. Hold either position for 60 seconds. Numbness and tingling in the thumb and first three fingers suggests compression of the median nerve due to the *carpal tunnel syndrome.*

● **Tinel's sign**: this is performed on one wrist after the other with the elbow flexed to about 90°, with the hand in the supine position, and the forearm, wrist and fingers in a straight line. Percuss lightly over the median nerve on the anterior surface of the wrist. Tingling or feelings of electricity suggest the *carpal tunnel syndrome.*

Spine

The patient should be standing for this.

Inspection

From the *front*:

● Observe the patient's posture, including the position of his trunk and neck and the erectness of his head. Fixed lateral flexion of the neck suggests *torticollis*, that is, spasm of the muscles in the neck that may be due to any of several causes.

From the *side*:

● Ask the patient to cover his front, expose his entire back and stand with his feet together and his arms by his sides.

● Assess any kyphosis or lordosis. *Kyphosis* is defined as an abnormal anterior *concavity* of the thoracic spine; *lordosis* is defined as an abnormal anterior *convexity* of the lumbar spine.

From *behind*:

● Look for *scoliosis* or tilt of the pelvis. Normally, a line between the two shoulders and another between the two iliac crests are parallel to one another. Sloped alignment suggests scoliosis or tilt of the pelvis.

Differentiating between true scoliosis and a shortened leg

● Note whether the pelvis appears to be horizontal. A shortened leg will cause the pelvis to tilt down on the side of the shortening and result in the spine adopting a scoliotic position. A true scoliosis will also cause the pelvis to tilt, but in this case, to compensate for the tilt, as the two legs are of equal length, *the hip and the knee will be slightly flexed on the side on which the pelvis is lowest.*

Palpation

- **Neck:** palpate the *facet joints*, first on one side and then the other, as they lie between the cervical vertebrae at a distance of approximately 2–3 cm lateral to the midline.

- **Whole spine:** in the midline, palpate the spinous processes of each vertebra with your thumb. Tenderness suggests injury, infection, dislocation or malignancy.

- **Lumbar spine:** in the lower lumbar area, apart from palpating for tenderness, also palpate for *spondylolisthesis*, which is a 'step' suggestive of forward displacement of one vertebra upon another; this is most commonly L4 upon L5, but also L5 upon the body of the sacrum. Forward displacement of one vertebra upon another may occasionally lead to compression of the spinal cord.

- **Sacroiliac joints:** palpate the sacroiliac joints, often identifiable by a dimple immediately inferior to the posterior superior iliac spine.

- The **vertebral muscles:** palpate the vertebral muscles on either side of the spine for tenderness or spasm.

Percussion

- Percuss the spine for tenderness by gently thumping with the ulnar surface of your fist. Pain on percussion may be due to osteoporosis, infection or malignancy of the underlying bones.

Sciatic nerve

- Ask the patient to lie on one side and flex his hips and knees, so you can palpate the sciatic nerve on the uppermost side. To do this, palpate the greater tuberosity and the greater trochanter. The greater trochanter is the bony prominence at the lateral upper end of the femur, and the greater tuberosity is the bony lower extremity of the pelvis that is to be felt on the *medial side* of the back of the upper thigh. The nerve lies half way between these two structures as it exits the pelvis via the sciatic notch. Tenderness over the nerve suggests a herniated disc or a pathological mass impinging on it in the pelvis.

● Finally, ask the patient to turn over, and repeat the test on the opposite side.

Range of motion of the neck

● **Flexion:** ask the patient to put his chin on his chest. Normally the range is 45°.

● **Extension:** ask the patient to look up at the ceiling and then backwards as far as he can. Normally, the range is 70°.

● **Rotation:** ask the patient to turn his head laterally as far as he can, first to one side and then to the other. Normally, the range is 70°.

● **Lateral bending:** ask the patient to tilt his head as far as he can towards his shoulder, first on one side, then on the other. Normally, the range is 40°.

Range of motion of the remaining spine

● **Flexion:** ask the patient to bend forward and touch his toes while keeping his legs straight. Normally, the range is 40–90°. Persistence of any lumbar lordosis in the flexed position suggests muscle spasm or, occasionally in a young man, *ankylosing spondylitis*.

Note!

The next three tests (extension, rotation and lateral bending) are performed with you standing behind the patient and steadying his pelvis by gripping it on both sides with your hands. The range of rotation is the movement before the pelvis begins to move.

- **Extension**: Ask the patient to bend his spine backwards as far as possible without moving his pelvis. Normally, the range is 30°.

- **Rotation**: Ask the patient to rotate the upper part of his trunk as far as he can without twisting his pelvis, first to one side then to the other. Normally, the range is 30°.

- **Lateral bending**: Ask the patient to bend laterally as far as he can without moving his pelvis, first to one side and then to the other. Normally, the range is 35°.

Note!

Limited motion of the neck and remaining spine may be due to arthritis such as osteoarthritis or ankylosing spondylitis, trauma, infection, malignancy or, in the case of the neck, muscle spasm due to torticollis. In the lower spine, limited motion may be due to herniation of an intervertebral disc, typically between L4/L5 or L5/S1.

Legs

Unless the patient has an injury to the legs, he should initially be standing upright with his feet together.

General inspection

- **Congenital deformities of the knee**: note whether there is *genu varum* (knees separated when the patient is standing with his feet together – 'bow legs'), or *genu valgum* (feet separated when the patient is standing with his knees together – 'knock knees').

- **Gait**: if you have not already observed the patient's gait, ask him to walk up and down in front of you, noticing his posture and the way he swings his arms and moves his feet. A description of several abnormal gaits is on page 39.

Hip

Inspection. To assess the hip for hidden fixed flexion deformity (usually due to osteoarthritis):

● Ask the patient to lie in the supine position.

● On lying flat, a patient with a fixed flexion deformity of the hip may compensate and keep his leg straight on the examination table by arching his spine and adopting a lordotic position.

● This can be eliminated and the back rendered straight on the table and the flexion deformity exposed by asking the patient to flex the opposite hip and knee. In the presence of a fixed flexion deformity, the femur on the affected side will rise a little and the knee on that side will visibly flex and rise a few centimetres.

To assess the length and symmetry of the legs (a test performed on both legs):

● Ask the patient to lie 'squarely,' so that an imaginary line between the iliac crests is at right angles to the line of the spine and both legs if possible.

● Assess the symmetry of the legs, and use a tape measure to measure the distance from the anterior superior iliac spine to the *medial* malleolus. Differences in the length of the legs are seen with a shortened leg, abduction and adduction deformities and fracture of the neck of the femur.

Note!

Due to contraction of the iliopsoas muscle, the length of the femoral neck and the way the muscle is inserted onto the femur, the leg is characteristically shortened and externally rotated with a fracture of the neck of the femur.

Palpation. This is carried out on one hip after the other.

With the patient still supine, palpate as follows:

- **Along the inguinal ligament**: bulges along the ligament may be due to an inguinal hernia, enlarged lymph nodes or, rarely, an aneurysm of the femoral artery.

- **Iliopectineal (or iliopsoas) bursa**: this bursa lies over the front of the hip joint and iliopsoas muscle, lateral to the femoral artery. Inflammation of the bursa is an unusual cause of pain in the hip.

- **Trochanteric bursa**: this bursa lies superficially over the greater trochanter on the lateral side of the upper end of the femur.

- **Ischiogluteal bursa**: this bursa is superficial to the ischial tuberosity, which is located at the top of the medial side of the back of the thigh. The patient will need to lie on his side with his hips and knees flexed in order for you to palpate it.

Range of motion. This is performed on both legs with the patient in the supine position.

Flexion is tested first on one side and then on the other:

- Ask the patient to bend his knee and bring it up to his chest, pulling it firmly against his abdomen. Normally, the range is 120°.

Extension is tested on one side and then the other:

- Ask the patient to turn over onto his abdomen and relax.

- Now gently grasp the lower front of the thigh and extend it backwards. Normally, the range is limited.

Abduction and *adduction* are tested on one side, and then the test is repeated on the other side.

For *abduction*:

- Ask the patient to return to the supine position. Anchor his pelvis by pressing down lightly on one of his anterior superior iliac spines with your left hand. Then, with your right hand, gently grasp the lower part of the opposite leg and abduct it until you feel the iliac spine begin to move. Normally, the range is 70°.

Adduction:

● While the patient is still supine and you are gripping the lower part of his leg and anchoring his pelvis, move the leg medially so that it crosses the other leg. Normally, the range is limited.

Rotation is tested first on one side and then on the other:

● Ask the patient to bend both his knee and his hip by 90°, so that his thigh is vertical and his lower leg is horizontal, as demonstrated in Fig. 16.6. Anchor the knee with your left hand and grasp the lower part of the leg with your right hand. Now rotate the lower part of the leg medially for external rotation and laterally for internal rotation. Normally, external rotation is 40° and internal rotation is 45°.

● Restricted flexion, abduction, external and internal rotation are common signs of osteoarthritis of the hip.

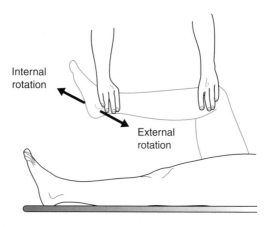

Fig 16.6 Rotation of the hip

Knee

Inspection

- With the patient still lying in the supine position, perform all of the following inspections on one side and then on the other.

- Check the alignment and contours of the knee, noting any injury, misalignment, swelling or redness

- **Patella**: inspect the patella for swelling and redness suggestive of inflammation of the prepatellar bursa, known as *housemaid's knee.*

- **Suprapatellar pouch**: inspect the area superior to the patella, noting any swelling suggestive of synovial thickening or effusion.

- **Areas adjacent to the patella**: note any loss of the normal hollows at the sides of the patella suggestive of swelling due to synovial thickening or effusion.

Palpation

For the *prepatellar bursa*, palpate first one side then the other:

- While the patient is still supine and the leg is extended, palpate the front of the patella for swelling and tenderness suggestive of inflammation of the prepatellar bursa, which, as mentioned above, is known as *housemaid's knee.*

For the *popliteal fossa*:

- Palpate behind the knee with the fingers of both hands for a swelling indicative of either a Baker's cyst, which is a backward protrusion of the capsule of the knee joint, or a pulsatile swelling suggestive of an aneurysm of the popliteal artery.

The *suprapatellar pouch* is palpated first on one side and then on the other:

- Palpate the area superior to the patella, noting any swelling or tenderness.

The remaining structures of the knee are then palpated:

● Ask the patient to flex his hip and knee, but keep his foot on the examination table.

● Cup your hands round the upper part of his calf with your thumbs in front and your fingers behind, and palpate the following three structures on one leg and then on the other.

● **Tibial tuberosity:** use your thumbs to palpate the tibial tuberosity lying in the middle of the top of the tibia, and the patellar tendon, which runs from the tibial tuberosity to the patella.

● **Tibial plateaux:** use your thumbs to palpate the medial and lateral tibial plateaux, which are located at the extreme top of the tibia on either side of the tibial tuberosity. Irregular bony ridges suggest osteoarthritis.

● **Menisci:** use your thumbs to palpate the medial and lateral menisci in the soft areas above the tibial plateaux, *immediately* on either side of the patella tendon. Tenderness suggests a torn meniscus (more common with the medial meniscus).

● **Special test for the menisci:** if you suspect a torn meniscus, perform *McMurray's test* by asking the patient to flex both his hip and knee to 90° so that the thigh is vertical and the lower part of the leg is horizontal, as it was for demonstrating rotation of the hip. Now steady the patient's knee with your left hand and place your right hand on his lower tibia. Twist the tibia so that the toes turn medially, and slowly extend the leg to investigate the lateral meniscus; then repeat the test but twist the tibia laterally to investigate the medial meniscus. Pain on twisting suggests a damaged or torn meniscus.

Detection of fluid in the knee joint. This is performed with the leg extended straight out on the examination table.

Bulge sign

● Part the thumb and index finger of your left hand and place the web between them over the upper part of the suprapatellar pouch above the knee. Gently squeeze from the top downwards to 'milk' any fluid from the pouch into the main part of the joint.

● While still maintaining pressure on the suprapatellar pouch, use the index finger or thumb of your right hand to apply pressure to the medial side of the joint and force any fluid over to the lateral side.

● Remove your right index finger or thumb and use it to tap any fluid that has been forced over to the lateral side of the joint. A bulge appearing on the medial side indicates fluid in the knee.

Balloon sign

● Without exerting pressure, lightly place the web between the thumb and index finger of your left hand over the upper part of the suprapatellar pouch above the knee.

● Now place the thumb and index finger of your right hand in the hollows that are normally on either side of the knee joint.

● Exert pressure with your *left* hand and 'milk' any fluid downwards from the suprapatellar pouch. Fluid is present if the fingers of your right hand are forced further apart.

Patellar tap (for large effusions)

● Place the web between the thumb and index finger of your left hand over the suprapatellar pouch above the knee and gently squeeze from the top downwards to 'milk' any fluid from the pouch into the main part of the joint.

● While still maintaining pressure on the suprapatellar pouch, place the index and middle fingers of your right hand on the patella, and then push them smartly down to strike the patella against the femur. A palpable tap indicates that fluid has lifted the patella away from the femur. Normally, the two bones are so closely applied to one another that a tap does not occur.

Assessment of painful ligaments. With the patient still supine and his leg initially extended straight out on the examination table, test the medial and lateral collateral ligaments on one knee and then the other. Then test the anterior and posterior cruciate ligaments on one side and then the other.

Medial and lateral collateral ligaments

- Palpate the medial and lateral collateral ligaments on either side of the knee.

- Now gently grasp and steady the lower part of the thigh with your left hand, and take hold of the lower part of the leg with your right hand. Try to move it laterally to test the medial ligament and medially to test the lateral ligament.

Note!

Tenderness on palpation or pain and displacement of the lower part of leg when an attempt is made to move it occur with damage or tears of the ligaments.

Anterior cruciate ligament (the anterior drawer sign)

- Ask the patient to bend his hip and knee, but keep his foot on the examination table.

- Cup your hands round the upper part of his calf with your thumbs in front and your fingers behind. Now gently pull the lower part of the leg forward. Forward movement of the lower part of the leg on the upper part that causes the contours of the tibial plateau to be exposed (like a drawer sliding forwards) occurs with rupture of the anterior cruciate ligament (so named because it is inserted into the anterior part of the tibial plateaux).

Posterior cruciate ligament (the posterior drawer sign)

● While maintaining your grip, gently try to push the lower part of the leg backwards. Backward movement of the lower part of the leg on the upper part (like a drawer sliding backwards) occurs with rupture of the posterior cruciate ligament.

Range of motion. Test this first on one side and then on the other.

● Ask the patient to straighten his leg on the table and then flex his hip to 90° so he can flex his knee as far as possible. Normally, the knee flexes to 120°.

Ankle and foot

This is performed with the patient in the supine position.
Inspection – on one side then on the other.

● Inspect the ankles and feet noting any redness, swelling, deformities, calluses or corns. Redness and swelling of the proximal joint of the big toe are common with gout

Palpation. Palpate all the following structures on one foot and then on the other.

● **Ankle:** use both hands for this particular part of the examination.

● Place your thumbs on either side of the front of the joint and your fingers on its sides, and palpate the ankle joint and its ligaments, noting any swelling, bogginess, tenderness or abnormal lateral or medial movements suggestive of torn lateral or medial ligaments.

● **Achilles tendon:** with the fingers and thumb of one hand, palpate the Achilles tendon for rheumatoid nodules, tendonitis, bursitis and tears.

● **Heel:** palpate the heel, in particular feeling the posterior and inferior surfaces of the calcaneus (Fig. 16.7) and the plantar fascia for tenderness and bony spurs:

● **Metatarsals:** arch your right hand immediately above the mid-foot, and use your fingers and thumb to palpate the metatarsal bones as a group (Fig. 16.7). Tenderness may be due to injury or arthritis.

● **Metatarsophalangeal joints and toes:** palpate each metatarsophalangeal joint with your thumb on top and your index finger underneath, and then palpate each toe. Tenderness occurs with trauma and arthritis. Tenderness of the big toe is common with gout.

Range of motion. Perform all the following tests on one foot and then the other.

● **Dorsiflexion and plantarflexion:** ask the patient to first dorsiflex and then plantarflex (extend) his foot as far as possible. Normally, dorsiflexion is 20° and plantarflexion is 45°.

● **Subtalar or talocalcaneal joint:** grasp and stabilize the lower leg at the ankle with your right hand.

● Now grasp the heel with your left hand and first invert and then evert the foot. Normally, inversion is 30° and eversion is 20°.

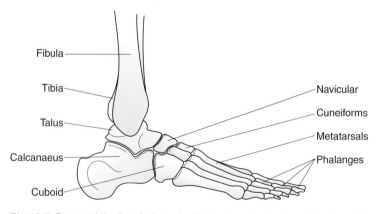

Fig 16.7 Bones of the foot (adapted with kind permission from Abrahams P, Craven J and Lumley J, *Illustrated Clinical Anatomy*, Great Britain: Hodder Education, 2005)

- Pain occurs with arthritis. Pain on stretching the lateral ligament by both inverting and plantarflexing the foot at the same time occurs with damage of the lateral ligament, that is, with a sprained ankle.

- **Transverse tarsal–metatarsal joint**: grasp the heel with your left hand to stabilize the proximal foot.

- Now grasp the metatarsals with your right hand, and first invert and then evert the distal part of the foot.

- **Metatarsophalangeal joints**: ask the patient to dorsiflex and plantarflex his toes. Normally, the big toe has a good range of motion.

17

BREASTS AND AXILLAE

Equipment needed

- None

Order of the examination

- Inspection
- Palpation

Position of the patient

- The patient should be sitting upright and wearing a robe in warm, quiet surroundings

Note!

Some clinicians prefer to examine the breasts and axillae at the end of the examination of the respiratory system.

EXAMINATION

Female breast

This is performed on both breasts.

> ## Note!
>
> If possible, the breasts should be examined after menstruation, as they are less tender and sensitive then.

Inspection

● Ask the patient to bare the upper part of her body and expose her breasts.

● Inspect the breasts with the arms in at least the first three of the four following positions:
  ○ with the arms by the sides
  ○ with the arms raised above the head
  ○ with the elbows flexed and the hands pressed against the hips
  ○ finally, if the breasts are large and pendulous, with the patient leaning forwards, so that the breasts hang free from the body.

● Look for changes in the skin and the size, symmetry and contours of each breast, and the nipples for the changes described in the paragraph titled *Nipple*.

Skin changes

● Redness may reflect underlying inflammation such as an infection or a carcinoma.

● Thickening or dimpling of the skin or prominence of the pores of the skin may also reflect an underlying carcinoma.

Size and symmetry

● Some difference in the size of the breasts and areolae of the nipples is normal. A large difference should arouse suspicion of a mass such as a carcinoma, or uncommonly, an abscess.

Contours

● Visible masses or flattening of the normal convexity of the breast should arouse suspicion of an underlying cancer.

Nipples

- Occasionally, the nipples are naturally inverted or depressed below the surrounding areola. However, any *recent change*, such as a discharge, change of shape, retraction of a nipple or an eczematous, scaly encrusted condition of the nipple known as *Paget's disease*, should arouse suspicion of an underlying carcinoma,

Palpation

This is also performed on both breasts.

- Ask the patient to lie in the supine position with the arm on the side to be examined raised over her head.

- Gently compress the breast against the chest wall with the *pads* of your fingers, using small rotatory movements to apply light, medium and deep pressure while performing whichever of the following patterns you feel most comfortable with:
  - working out from the centre in radial lines like the hands of a clock in a quadrant by quadrant manner
  - in concentric circles, starting either in the centre working outwards, or in the periphery working inwards, in which case you will end up ready to examine the nipple
  - in horizontal parallel lines, starting at the top and working downwards
  - finally, having palpated the main part of the breast, carefully palpate its tail, which lies towards the axilla.

- Check the consistency of the breast, noting any masses, or tenderness such as sometimes occurs premenstrually.

Masses

- Palpate and note the size, shape and consistency of any mass, that is, whether it is hard or soft, smooth or irregular, or poorly circumscribed. Also note whether it is attached to the skin or fixed to the underlying pectoral muscles.

- A hard, irregular, poorly circumscribed mass that is attached to the skin or deep tissues strongly suggests a carcinoma.

Nipple

- Note the consistency of the nipple and whether palpation results in a discharge. Thickening or loss of elasticity of the nipple or a bloody discharge should arouse suspicion of a carcinoma.

Inspection of the axillae

This is done for both men and women, and should be performed on both sides.

- The patient should be either sitting or lying supine. In either case, ask the patient to raise one arm so that the axilla may be inspected.

- Inspect the skin of the axilla, noting any rashes caused by deodorant or fungal infection, infection of the sweat glands or unusual pigmentation such as *acanthosis nigrans*, which is a smooth, velvety, raised brown or almost black rash that is occasionally seen in obese persons and also as an external marker of internal malignancy or endocrine disease such as diabetes mellitus.

Palpation of the axillae

- Three groups of lymph nodes are palpated from the front. These are the *central nodes,* the *pectoral nodes* and the *lateral nodes.* A fourth group, the *subscapular nodes* are palpated from behind the patient.

- To accomplish palpation of the first three groups, the patient should be sitting with the arm to be examined slightly flexed, abducted and supported by one of your hands, so that your right hand is free to examine the patient's left side and your left hand is free to examine the right side.

- **Central nodes**: cup your fingers and place their tips as high up in the axilla as possible; then run them down the lateral wall of the chest, feeling for any swelling.

- **Pectoral nodes**: grasp the pectoral fold with your thumb in front and your index and middle fingers behind, and palpate the pectoral nodes on the back of the pectoral fold.

- **Lateral nodes**: cup your fingers and place their tips high up on the lateral wall of the axilla; feel for nodes as you sweep down the medial side of the upper part of the humerus.

- **Subscapular nodes**: position yourself behind the patient. Place your thumb behind and your index and middle fingers in front of the posterior axillary fold, and palpate the subscapular nodes on the front of the fold.

MALE BREAST

Examination is performed on both breasts.

Inspection

- Inspect the breasts for size, symmetry and contours.

- Enlargement of the breast may be due to obesity, in which case it is soft, or gynaecomastia, due for instance to liver disease, in which case it is firmer.

- Inspect the nipples and areolae for nodules and ulceration.

Palpation

- Palpate the breasts and nipples with the *pads* of your fingers, noting any masses. Carcinoma of the male breast occasionally occurs.

18

FEMALE GENITALIA AND RECTAL EXAMINATION

Equipment needed

- Bright light on a stand
- Vaginal specula of various sizes
- Materials for cervical smears, i.e. glass microscope slides, slide covers, cotton swabs, cervical spatula and brushes, spray-can of fixative
- Microscope
- Culture media for *Neisseria gonorrhoeae*, *Chlamydia trachomatis* and other bacterial and fungal infections, or a nucleic acid probe test kit for identifying *Neisseria gonorrhoeae* and *Chlamydia trachomatis*
- Gloves
- Water-soluble lubricant
- pH paper, a small bottle of potassium hydroxide solution and another of normal saline
- Tissues.

Note about gloves

Practice varies concerning gloves. Some clinicians glove both hands; others glove their non-dominant hand and use the other hand for handling instruments; others glove the dominant hand; still others double-glove one hand. In view of this, it is suggested that you follow the practice in your institution, remembering to use only a gloved hand when touching the patient's genitalia.

Position of the patient

- The patient should have emptied her bladder.
- Ask her to lie in the dorsal position, that is, supine on the examination table with her hips flexed and abducted, her knees flexed, and her feet flat and apart on the corners of the leading edge of the table.

    Alternatively, if it is the practice in your institution, ask her to lie in the lithotomy position with her hips flexed and abducted, her knees flexed and her feet resting in foot-rests.

- Then cover her legs and abdomen with drapes, leaving only the perineum visible.

Keeping the patient informed

Inform the patient each time **before** touching her or doing anything to her. Also remember to be accompanied by a chaperone, and to be gentle and avoid making personal comments.

EXAMINATION (INITIALLY EXTERNALLY)

- Glove your hand(s) and seat yourself so that you are facing the patient's perineum.

Box 18.1: Checklist of structures to be inspected

External examination
- Mons pubis
- Labia majora and minora
- Clitoris, immediately inferior to the superior folds of the labia minora
- Urethral meatus, immediately inferior to the clitoris
- Vaginal opening or introitus
- Bartholin's glands on either side of the inferior aspect of the vaginal opening
- Perineum

Internal examination
- Vaginal walls
- Cervix
- Uterus, ovaries and adnexae
- Pelvic muscles
- Rectovaginal wall
- Anus and rectum

Inspection and palpation

- **Inspect the mons pubis** (the prominence formed by the fat pad over the pubic area) for hair distribution, nits, lice, folliculitis and excoriation.

- **Inspect the labia majora and minora** looking for bruising, swelling, ulcers or nodules.

- **Inspect the perineum and perianal areas** looking for lumps, ulcers, inflammation, rashes or haemorrhoids. If present, fistulae or abscesses are suggestive of Crohn's disease or diverticular disease.

- **Inspection of the clitoris, urethral meatus, Bartholin's glands and vaginal opening (introitus):** warn the patient you are about to touch her, and, using your gloved hand, gently part the labia minora and inspect the clitoris, urethral meatus, Bartholin's glands and vaginal opening,

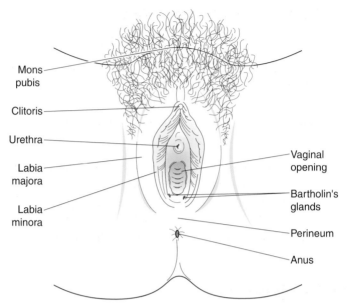

Mons pubis

Clitoris

Urethra

Labia majora

Labia minora

Vaginal opening

Bartholin's glands

Perineum

Anus

Fig 18.1 Female genitalia (adapted from Luesley D, *Common Conditions in Gynaecology*, (1998). London: Chapman and Hall. By kind permission of the author)

looking for inflammation, ulcers, bruising, discharge, swelling and nodules.

Palpation of Bartholin's glands

● Place your thumb outside and your index finger inside the vaginal entrance and feel posterolaterally, repeating on the other side. Swelling suggests a Bartholin's cyst; swelling plus tenderness suggests infection of the gland.

Internal examination

This is performed with you sitting.

Initial identification of the cervix, using one finger

● Lubricate the index finger of your gloved hand with water (other lubricants may spoil any specimens you take) and gently insert it into the vagina. Identify the firm, rounded surface of the cervix with the tip of your finger (it feels like the tip of your nose).

Checking for urethritis and urethral discharge

● Position your hand so that the palm is facing upwards and the palmar surface of your index finger is against the anterior surface of the vagina. Now slowly withdraw your hand and 'milk' the urethra with the tip of your finger. Culture or use the DNA test kit to test any discharge for *Neisseria gonorrhoeae* and *Chlamydia trachomatis.*

Vaginal walls and rectocoele

● Remove your finger, separate the labia with your index and middle fingers and ask the patient to bear down. Note any bulging of the vaginal walls suggestive of a cystocoele (an abnormal bulge of the anterior vaginal wall) or rectocoele (an abnormal bulge of the posterior vaginal wall).

Speculum examination

Insertion of the speculum

● Take hold of the speculum in your ungloved hand with your index and middle fingers surrounding the blades, as if holding a cigarette. Place your fourth and fifth fingers over the back of the handle with your thumb resting on the moveable front of the handle. Now lubricate the speculum with water.

● Open the introitus by inserting your gloved index finger or both your index and middle fingers into the vagina, and gently press down on the posterior wall towards the anus/rectum. This will relax the deep pelvic floor.

● Advise the patient that you are about to insert the speculum. Then, aiming backwards and slightly downwards towards the rectum to avoid hurting the anterior structures, insert the speculum over your fingers with its blades at an angle of 45° to the vertical, twisting it as it enters so that the trigger for opening it ends up pointing downwards. Remember to look down into the vagina as you insert the instrument, and to be careful not to hurt the patient. Finally, withdraw your fingers.

Inspection of the cervix

● Open the speculum carefully, and find and inspect the cervix, noting its position, surfaces, the os and any ulceration, nodules, masses, bleeding or discharge.

Obtaining specimens for cervical cytology (Pap smear)

● Take an **endocervical** specimen by partially inserting a cervical brush or cotton swab into the os of the cervix, but use only a cotton swab on pregnant patients.

● Take an **ectocervical** specimen by placing the long arm of a spatula in the os and then sweeping round the os with the short arm for 360°.

● Immediately after taking each specimen, and before it dries, gently spread it on an appropriately labelled slide and fix it.

Inspection of the vagina and withdrawal of the speculum

● Unlock the speculum and slowly withdraw it. At the same time, rotate it through 45°, so that the blades are withdrawn at an angle of 45° to the vertical. In this way, you will avoid hurting the patient. As you withdraw the speculum, inspect the walls of the vagina, noting their colour and any inflammation, discharge, ulcers or masses.

● **Oedema and redness** of the vaginal wall are specific indications of infection with *Trichomonas vaginalis.*

● A **white curdy discharge** in the vagina is suggestive of, but not specific for, infection with *Candida albicans* (*Monilia*).

● A **yellow discharge** is suggestive of, but not specific for, infection with either *bacteria* or *Trichomonas vaginalis.*

Vaginal specimens (taken if indicated by the presence of a discharge or because of local practice)

● As you withdraw the speculum, use either a Q-tip dipped in saline or the nucleic acid probe test kit to take specimens for culturing or testing for *Neisseria gonorrhoeae* or *Chlamydia trachomatis.*

- Dip another Q-tip in saline and gently rub it on the vaginal wall to take a sample of vaginal or cervical mucous for a wet smear and pH test.

- Gently roll the second Q-tip on a microscope slide and immediately inspect the sample under a microscope. Small, round, semi-transparent moving bodies indicate infection with *Trichomonas vaginalis.*

- Clue cells, which are superficial epithelial vaginal cells whose crisp outlines have been obscured by millions of adherent bacteria, are seen under the microscope with bacterial infections.

- Remove the slide from the microscope and add one drop of potassium hydroxide. A fishy smell occurs in about two-thirds of cases of infection with *Trichomonas vaginalis*, but the test is negative with monilial infection.

- Again, inspect the slide under the microscope. The potassium hydroxide lyses all cellular material except fungi, which are therefore visible, enabling a diagnosis of fungal infection to be made.

- Now rub the Q-tip on a pH paper. The pH of the healthy vagina is normally less than 4.5; with bacterial or trichomonal infections it becomes alkaline; and with monilial infection it is usually normal, that is, under 4.5.

Box 18.2: Clinical features of pregnancy

Symptoms
- Amenorrhoea (i.e. missed period)
- Morning sickness (one of the first symptoms)
- Breast enlargement with tingling around the nipples from about 6 weeks
- Urinary frequency from about 6 weeks
- Weight gain
- Increased risk of diabetes
- Increased risk of pulmonary embolus (page 136)
- Risk of toxaemia

Signs
- Mild tachycardia, increased pulse volume
- Fundus, palpable:
  - *12 weeks*: above the pubic bone
  - *16 weeks*: midway between the pubic bone and the umbilicus
  - *20 weeks*: lower border of the umbilicus
  - *28 weeks*: midway between the umbilicus and the xiphisternum
  - *34 weeks*: just below the xiphisternum
- Breasts larger and warmer than normal with visible veins, darkening of the areolae and development of Montgomery's tubercles

Bimanual examination (palpation)

This is performed with you standing.

- Lubricate the index and middle fingers of your gloved hand with lubricant and slide them into the vagina, remembering to keep your thumb away from the sensitive clitoris. (If both your hands are gloved, you may facilitate this procedure by opening the introitus and holding the posterior wall of the vagina down with the index finger of your other hand, as you did when inserting the speculum.)

- Palpate the posterior, lateral and anterior walls of the vagina, noting any tenderness or nodularity. Stool in the rectum may be felt through the posterior vaginal wall.

- Now turn your hand so that the palmar surface is facing upwards, and palpate the anterior part of the vagina in the vicinity of the urethra and bladder.

- **Definitive palpation of the cervix**: palpate the cervix, feeling its position, shape, consistency and mobility, and any tenderness suggestive of pelvic inflammatory disease.

- **Palpation of the uterus**: first place your ungloved hand on the abdomen above the pubic symphysis (your gloved hand is already in the vagina). Now, for support, stand with the elbow of the hand that is in the vagina against your trunk and lift the cervix, at the same time pressing in gently with the hand on the pubis symphysis to grasp the uterus between your two hands. Note its shape, size and consistency. Enlargement of the uterus suggests pregnancy, fibroids, malignant tumour or cysts.

● Bimanually palpate laterally on either side of the uterus to identify the ovaries, feeling for their size and any tumours, cysts, swelling or tenderness. At the same time, feel for the adjacent adnexa (i.e. the Fallopian tubes, round and broad ligaments), although normally they are not palpable.

Box 18.3: The symptoms and signs of impending eclampsia (convulsion related to pregnancy)

● Have a high index of suspicion, particularly in any pregnant woman with a high blood pressure (diastolic >90 mmHg) and proteinuria

Symptoms
● Unusual headache
● Visual disturbance
● Agitation or restlessness
● Upper abdominal pain, nausea or vomiting

Signs
● Fluid retention and poor urinary output causing weight gain and oedema
● Hyperreflexia or ankle clonus (page 210)
● Retinal haemorrhages, oedema or papilloedema (pages 186 and 182)

Amended from Drife J, Magowan BA. *Clinical Obstetrics and Gynaecology*. Elsevier, 2004: 372.

● **Assessing the strength of the pelvic floor muscles:** do this by slowly withdrawing and spreading your fingers against the vaginal walls at the same time as asking the patient to squeeze your fingers with the muscles of her pelvic floor. Age, vaginal deliveries and neurological deficits may contribute to weakness, which may also be associated with stress incontinence. Complete the withdrawal of your fingers.

- **Rectovaginal examination**: change your glove or peel off one glove if you are double-gloved. Advise the patient that you are about to examine both her vagina and rectum. Then place the *pad* (not the tip) of the *middle finger* of your gloved hand pointing anteriorly on the anal sphincter to allow it to relax.

- Gently insert the finger into the rectum and note whether the anal canal is abnormally lax or abnormally tight, suggesting anal stenosis. At the same time, insert the *index finger* of the same hand into the vagina.

- Then, with your other hand placed above the pubic symphysis, repeat the bimanual examination to palpate the uterus and identify whether it is retroverted. In addition, use the finger in the rectum to feel the space behind the cervix

---

Box 18.4: Clinical features of acute salpingitis

Symptoms
- Unwellness, bilateral lower abdominal pain, vomiting ± constipation, dehydration
- Vaginal discharge

Signs
- Fever
- Bilateral lower abdominal tenderness ± rebound tenderness, possibly leading to peritonitis and abdominal distension and rigidity
- Vaginal discharge
- Pelvic examination: pain in the fornices plus tenderness of the uterus, particularly on manipulation

- **Rectal examination**: remove your index finger from the vagina and use your middle finger (which is already in the rectum) to perform a rectal examination, sweeping it first round 180° in a clockwise direction and then 360° in an anticlockwise direction to feel for any tenderness, induration or masses. The cervix is often palpable anteriorly and may be mistaken for a mass.

- Remove your finger from the rectum and note any blood; if none is visible, test any faecal matter for occult blood and, if necessary, send a specimen for bacterial culture.

- Finally, either clean the anus yourself or give the patient some tissues to do so.

Box 18.5: Clinical features of polycystic ovary disease

Classically a triad of:
- Obesity
- Hirsutism
- Infertility with oligo/amenorrhoea

Other clinical features
- Acne and hirsutism, possibly resulting in shaving
- Insulin resistance

19

MALE GENITALIA, ANUS, RECTUM AND PROSTATE

Equipment needed

- Gloves and water-soluble lubricant
- Microscope slides and slide covers
- Culture media for *Neisseria gonorrhoeae* and *Chlamydia trachomatis*, bacterial and fungal infections, or a nucleic acid probe test kit for identifying *Neisseria gonorrhoeae* and *Chlamydia trachomatis*
- Torch
- Tissues

Note about gloves

A glove is worn for examining the rectum and prostate gland, but practice varies if only the genitalia are to be examined, some clinicians wearing gloves whereas others do not.

Order of the examination

- Inspection
- Palpation

> **Position of the patient**
>
> ● The patient should be either standing or lying in the supine position in warm, quiet surroundings. Note that the standing position is preferred for detecting hernias

EXAMINATION

Penis

Inspection

● Inspect the surface of the penis, including the prepuce (foreskin), looking for ulcers, masses, scars or inflammation.

● Check the skin around the base of the penis, looking for fungal infection, excoriation and inflammation suggesting scabies, and also check the pubic hairs for nits and lice.

● If the foreskin is present, retract it or ask the patient to do so. It is normal for smegma (a whitish, cheesy material) to be present. Inspect the glans for ulcers, masses, scars or inflammation. Note the location of the urethral meatus. Hypospadias is a congenital ventral displacement of the urethral meatus.

Palpation

● **Urethral discharge**: compress the glans between your thumb and index finger, and note any discharge. Normally, there is none. If the patient complains of discharge but there is none, ask him to 'milk' the shaft of the penis. Place any discharge on a glass slide for microscopy and take specimens for culture. Gonococcal discharge tends to be yellow and profuse, whereas non-gonococcal discharge tends to be scanty and white or clear.

● Palpate the shaft of the penis between your thumb and first two fingers, noting any induration or tenderness. Induration and tenderness along the ventral surface of the penis suggests infection, possibly in association with a urethral stricture or rarely a carcinoma.

Note!

- **Phimosis** is a tight foreskin that cannot be retracted over the glans.
- **Paraphimosis** is a tight foreskin that once retracted cannot be returned to its normal position.
- **Balanitis** is inflammation of the glans.

Scrotum

Inspection

- Inspect the front of the scrotum; then lift it and inspect its posterior surface, looking for any rashes, epidermoid cysts or rarely carcinoma.

- Note any swelling, lumps or veins.

Palpation

Examine first one side and then the other.

- Palpate the testes, epididymis and spermatic cord between your fingers and thumb.

- **Testes:** note the size of each testis and its shape, consistency and any tenderness. Normally, the testes are smooth, ovoid, sensitive to pressure and about 4–5 cm long.

- **Epididymis** is softer than the testis; it is located on the posterolateral surface of the testis.

- **Spermatic cord** may be palpated from the tail of the epididymis to the external inguinal ring. The cord contains blood vessels, nerves, muscle fibres and the vas deferens running from the tail of the epididymis to the inguinal canal and then via the pelvis to the urethra.

- Marked thickening of the tissues at the external inguinal ring may be due to an indirect inguinal hernia that has entered the scrotum.

Transillumination of a scrotal swelling

- Opinion about the value of this test is divided.

- Darken the room; then place a torch behind the scrotum and shine a beam of light through the swelling.

- If the swelling lights up with a pale red glow, it is fluid filled and likely to be a *hydroceole*; if it does not, it may be a varicoceole, an indirect hernia or a solid tumour.

> **Note!**
>
> Background information about abnormalities of the scrotum is on page 284.

Inguinal area

Examination is performed first on one side and then on the other.

- If you have not already palpated the inguinal area for lymph nodes as part of the examination of the peripheral vascular system, do so now by palpating along the inguinal ligament.

- Small, shotty glands may be felt in healthy people. Swollen, tender glands suggest infection. Hard, irregular enlargement that is deeply attached suggests metastases from a pelvic carcinoma. Rubbery enlargement suggests lymphoma.

Hernias

- Ask the patient to stand, as hernias are most easily demonstrated in the standing position.

Inguinal hernia

● Ask the patient to cough or bear down, and observe the inguinal region for any swelling.

● Now prepare to explore the inguinal canal using your *right* index finger for the patient's *right* side and your *left* index finger for the patient's *left* side.

● Invaginate loose scrotal skin with the tip of your finger and follow the spermatic cord up to the slit-like opening of the external inguinal ring, as demonstrated in Fig. 19.1.

● Now, with your finger at the external ring or in the inguinal canal, ask the patient to cough or strain down.

● Note any herniating mass that strikes your fingertip; normally, there is none. If you feel one, it is likely to be due to an *indirect* inguinal hernia.

● Remove your hand and place it slightly above the centre of the inguinal canal; ask the patient to cough or strain down to test for a *direct* inguinal hernia.

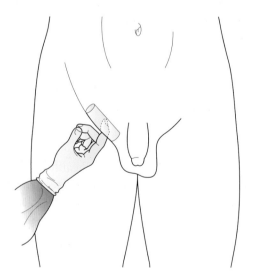

Fig 19.1 Examining the inguinal canal using invaginated scrotum

> **Note!**
>
> Background information about the different types of hernia is on page 281.

Femoral hernia

- First find the *femoral canal* lying beneath the inguinal ligament by palpating and identifying the pulsation of the femoral artery slightly to the medial side of the centre of the groin.

- *From medial to lateral*, the femoral canal contains three main structures, namely the femoral *vein*, the femoral *artery* and the femoral *nerve*, the order of which may be remembered by the word '*VAN*'.

- *Any hernia is medial to the femoral vein.*

- To check for a femoral hernia, first locate the femoral vein, medial to the pulsation of the femoral artery, and then place the pads of your fingers immediately medial to the vein; ask the patient to cough or strain down. Note any herniating mass or tenderness; normally, there is none.

Anus and rectum

This examination should be performed now if it has not already been performed as part of the examination of the abdomen.

Preparation

- Ask the patient to adopt the appropriate position.

- This is usually the *left lateral position*, with the patient lying on his left side with his knees and hips flexed.

- Occasionally, the examination is performed from behind with the patient standing and leaning over the examination table.

- Glove your right hand.

Perianal area

● Inspect and palpate the sacrococcygeal and perianal areas, noting any tenderness, lumps, ulcers, inflammation, rashes, haemorrhoids or pilonidal sinus (a short tract containing hairs that is prone to infection near the top of the natal cleft). If present, fistulae or abscesses are suggestive of Crohn's disease or diverticular disease.

Anus and rectum

● Lubricate your gloved index finger and advise the patient that you are about to place your finger on his anus.

● Lightly place the *pad* (not the tip) of your index finger pointing anteriorly on the anus, and after a few seconds the anal sphincter will relax.

● **Anal canal**: gently insert the finger into the anal canal, noting the tone of the sphincter and whether it is abnormally lax or is abnormally tight, suggesting anal stenosis. Also note any tenderness, induration or nodules.

● **Rectum**: enter your finger into the rectum and gently move it up as far as you can along the sacral hollow on the front of the sacrum.

● Sweep the walls of the rectum, first for 180° in a clockwise fashion, and then 360° in an anticlockwise fashion, noting any induration or masses suggestive of rectal carcinoma.

● **Prostate gland**: at the end of the anticlockwise or second sweep, withdraw your finger a little and examine the prostate gland lying anteriorly to the rectum.

● Palpate the posterior surface of the gland, noting both lateral lobes and the median sulcus between them. Normally, the prostate gland is rubbery and non-tender. The features of chronic prostatism are listed in Box 19.1.

Box 19.1: Clinical features of chronic prostatism

Urinary symptoms
- Frequency
- Urgency
- Hesitancy
- Poor/thin urinary stream
- Dribbling after micturition
- Nocturia more than once per night
- Risk of urinary infection due to urinary stasis
- Pain in the lower abdomen if urinary retention occurs

Signs
- Usually no abdominal signs
- Enlarged prostate on rectal examination
- Palpable bladder with urinary obstruction
- Signs of renal failure with longstanding obstruction

- Nodularity suggests cancer; tenderness suggests acute prostatitis due to bacterial infection (Box 19.2).

- Withdraw your finger from the rectum and note any blood. If there is none, test any faecal matter for occult blood.

- Finally, either clean the anus yourself or give the patient some tissues to do so.

Box 19.2: Clinical features of acute prostatitis

Symptoms
- Severe pain in the perineum

Signs
- Tenderness on pressure over the perineum
- Rectal examination: exquisite tenderness anteriorly over the prostate gland

BACKGROUND INFORMATION

Scrotum and hernias

Scrotum

- An **abnormally small scrotum** suggests an undescended testicle (*cryptorchidism*).

- A **swollen or enlarged** scrotum may be due to an *indirect inguinal* hernia, a *hydrocoele*, a *varicocoele*, a solid mass such as a *tumour*, or *oedema* of the scrotum secondary to right heart failure.

- A **hydrocoele** is a collection of fluid between the layers of the tunica vaginalis, which is a serous membrane surrounding the testis (except posteriorly).

- A **varicocoele** is abnormal congestion and dilatation of the spermatic vein within the scrotum, most commonly on the left side. This is because the vein on that side drains into the renal vein and is therefore longer than the vein on the right side; as a consequence, it is subject to higher hydrostatic back pressure.

- A **tender, swollen scrotum** occurs with acute epididymitis, acute orchitis, torsion of the spermatic cord or strangulated hernia.

Hernias

Ninety-five per cent of hernias in the groin are inguinal; the other five per cent are femoral.

- **Indirect inguinal hernia** emerges from the abdominal wall *lateral* to the inferior epigastric blood vessels and enters the inguinal canal at its lateral end through the deep inguinal ring.

- **Direct hernia** emerges from the abdominal wall at a point roughly half way along the back of the inguinal canal, *medial* to the inferior epigastric blood vessels.

CONCLUSION AND FURTHER READING

Having learned to take a history and examine a patient, one more thing remains to be done – practise, practise, practise. Apart from the rather abbreviated histories and physical examinations normally carried out in everyday clinical practice, try to take two or three *full* histories and to do one or two *full* examinations each week *throughout your training.*

It is, however, important not to fatigue or burden the patient. There are various way of achieving this. One is to ask a friend or colleague, instead of a patient, whether you can examine them. Another way is to go into greater than routine detail only with patients who are well enough, who understand what you are doing and who have given informed consent. A third way is to divide the large systems such as the musculoskeletal and nervous systems into parts such as the upper limb, or spine and cranial nerves, or motor system and, with the patient's consent, go into extra detail on just one part.

If you do these things or something similar on a regular basis, and if you read widely and readily embrace new ideas, you should become a well-rounded competent clinician and enjoy your work and help many people.

FURTHER READING

Bates B. *A Guide to Physical Examination and History Taking*, 8th edn. Lippincott; 2003.

Braunwald E, Zipes DP, Libby P, Bonow R. *Braunwald's Heart Disease: A Textbook of Cardiovascular Medicine*, 7th edn. WB Saunders; 2004.

Drife J, Magowan BA. *Clinical Obstetrics and Gynaecology*. Elsevier ; 2004. (First edition)

Floch MH, Floch NR, Kowdley KV. *Netter's Gastroenterology*. WB Saunders; 2004.

Hochberg MC, Silman AJ, Smolen JS, Weinblatt M, Weisman MH. *Rheumatology*, 3rd edn. Mosby; 2003.

Kanski JK. *Clinical Ophthalmology*, 5th edn. Butterworth Heinemann; 2003.

Pattern J. *Neurological Differential Diagnosis*, 2nd edn. Springer-Verlag; 2005.

Seaton AD, Leitch AG, Seaton D. *Crofton and Douglas's Respiratory Diseases*, 5th edn. Blackwell Science; 2000.

INDEX